Biologically Active Natural Products from Asia and Africa: A Selection of Topics

Edited by

Anna Capasso
Department of Pharmacy
University of Salerno, 84084 Fisciano SA
Italy

Biologically Active Natural Products from Asia and Africa:

A Selection of Topics

Editor: Anna Capasso

ISBN (Online): 978-981-14-8974-7

ISBN (Print): 978-981-14-8972-3

ISBN (Paperback): 978-981-14-8973-0

need for a court order if at any point you breach any terms of this License Agreement. In no event will any delay or failure by Bentham Science Publishers in enforcing your compliance with this License Agreement constitute a waiver of any of its rights.

3. You acknowledge that you have read this License Agreement, and agree to be bound by its terms and conditions. To the extent that any other terms and conditions presented on any website of Bentham Science Publishers conflict with, or are inconsistent with, the terms and conditions set out in this License Agreement, you acknowledge that the terms and conditions set out in this License Agreement shall prevail.

Bentham Science Publishers Pte. Ltd.
80 Robinson Road #02-00
Singapore 068898
Singapore
Email: subscriptions@benthamscience.net

BENTHAM SCIENCE

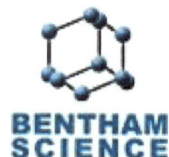

CONTENTS

Rausan Zamir, Nazmul Islam, Sunzid Ahmed, Md. Ali Asraf, Nikhil C. Bhoumik,
Omar Faruque and *Akhter Farooque*

Rausan Zamir, Nazmul Islam, Mahfuza Parveen, Shipra Sarker, Rajib Kanti,
M. Safiur Rahman and *Omar Faruque*

PREFACE

Both Asia and Africa have many plants that can be used for medicinal purposes: these medicinal plants are used in the treatment of many diseases and their uses and effects are of growing interest in western societies. Medicinal plants from Asia and Africa are not only used and chosen for their healing abilities, but also for a symbolic and spiritual meaning.

The importance of traditional autochthonous plant remedies plays a crucial role in the health of millions of people both in Asia and in Africa. Even today, traditional medicine represents the dominant medical system for millions of people showing a significant impact on health care practices. Therefore, traditional operators still represent a vital part of their health system. For this reason, even the pharmaceutical industries consider traditional medicine as a source for the identification of bioactive agents that can be used in the preparation of synthetic drugs.

This book will guide you to discover new natural products from Asia and Africa and the different ways to use them to treat or alleviate many of the most common diseases.

Anna Capasso
Department of Pharmacy
University of Salerno, 84084 Fisciano SA
Italy

List of Contributors

A. Zaifar	Faculty of Medicine, Universitas Indonesia, Jakarta, Indonesia
A.A. Yelmate	School of Pharmacy, S.R.T.M. University, Nanded, Maharashtra, India
Abdelhakim Bouyahya	Department of Biology, Faculty of Science, Genomic Center of Human Pathologies, Faculty of Medicine, Laboratory of Human Pathologies Biology, Mohammed V University, Rabat, Morocco
Akhter Farooque	Department of Chemistry, University of Rajshahi, Rajshahi, Bangladesh
Amina El Yahyaoui El Idrissi	Department of Biology, Faculty of Science, Genomic Center of Human Pathologies, Faculty of Medicine, Laboratory of Human Pathologies Biology, Mohammed V University, Rabat, Morocco
Aya Khouchlaa	Department of Biology, Faculty of Science, Genomic Center of Human Pathologies, Faculty of Medicine, Laboratory of Human Pathologies Biology, Mohammed V University, Rabat, Morocco
Charles O. Nnadi	Department of Pharmaceutical and Medicinal Chemistry, Faculty of Pharmaceutical Sciences, University of Nigeria Nsukka, 410001 Nsukka, Nigeria
Chigozie L. Ugwu	Department of Statistics, Faculty of Physical Sciences, University of Nigeria Nsukka, 410001 Nsukka, Nigeria
Chinwe M. Onah	Department of Pharmaceutical and Medicinal Chemistry, Faculty of Pharmaceutical Sciences, University of Nigeria Nsukka, 410001 Nsukka, Nigeria
E.N. Nabila	Faculty of Medicine, Universitas Indonesia, Jakarta, Indonesia
L.D. Vincent	Faculty of Medicine, Universitas Indonesia, Jakarta, Indonesia
M. Louisa	Department of Pharmacology and Therapeutics, Faculty of Medicine, Universitas Indonesia, Jakarta, Indonesia
M. Safiur Rahman	Atmospheric and Environmental Chemistry Laboratory, Chemistry Division, Atomic Energy Center, 4-Kazi Nazrul Islam Avenue, Dhaka-1000, Bangladesh
M'hamed Tijane	Department of Biology, Faculty of Science, Genomic Center of Human Pathologies, Faculty of Medicine, Laboratory of Human Pathologies Biology, Mohammed V University, Rabat, Morocco
Mahfuza Parveen	Department of Environmental Science and Disaster Management, Daffodil International University, Dhaka-1207, Bangladesh
Md. Ali Asraf	Department of Chemistry, University of Rajshahi, Rajshahi, Bangladesh
Md. Matiur Rahman	Department of Pharmacy, Ranada Prasad Shaha University, Narayanganj-1400, Bangladesh
Mereym El Fessikh	Department of Biology, Faculty of Science, Genomic Center of Human Pathologies, Faculty of Medicine, Laboratory of Human Pathologies Biology, Mohammed V University, Rabat, Morocco
Muhammad Torequl Islam	Department of Pharmacy, Life Science Faculty, Bangabandhu Sheikh Mujibur Rahman Science and Technology University, Gopalganj (Dhaka)-8100, Bangladesh
N.M.P Kusuma	Faculty of Medicine, Universitas Indonesia, Jakarta, Indonesia

Nazmul Islam	Department of General Educational Development, Daffodil International University, Dhaka, Bangladesh Department of Nutrition and Food Technology, Jashore University of Science and Technology, Jashore, Bangladesh
Nikhil C. Bhoumik	Wazed Miah Science Research Center, Jahangirnagar University, Savar, Dhaka, Bangladesh
Omar Faruque	Department of Nutrition and Food Technology, Jashore University of Science and Technology, Jashore, Bangladesh
P. Gundewar	School of Pharmacy, S.R.T.M. University, Nanded, Maharashtra, India
Pranta Ray	Department of Pharmacy, Life Science Faculty, Bangabandhu Sheikh Mujibur Rahman Science and Technology University, Gopalganj (Dhaka)-8100, Bangladesh
R.S. Moon	School of Pharmacy, S.R.T.M. University, Nanded, Maharashtra, India
Rajib Hossain	Department of Pharmacy, Life Science Faculty, Bangabandhu Sheikh Mujibur Rahman Science and Technology University, Gopalganj (Dhaka)-8100, Bangladesh
Rajib Kanti	Department of Nutrition and Food Technology, Jashore University of Science and Technology, Jashore, Bangladesh
Rausan Zamir	Department of Chemistry, University of Rajshahi, Rajshahi, Bangladesh
S.S.K. Nareswari	Department of Pharmacology and Therapeutics, Faculty of Medicine, Universitas Indonesia, Jakarta, Indonesia
Shipra Sarker	Department of Nutrition and Food Technology, Jashore University of Science and Technology, Jashore, Bangladesh
Sunzid Ahmed	Centre for Advanced Research in Science, University of Dhaka, Dhaka, Bangladesh
Wilfred O. Obonga	Department of Pharmaceutical and Medicinal Chemistry, Faculty of Pharmaceutical Sciences, University of Nigeria Nsukka, 410001 Nsukka, Nigeria
Youssef Bakri	Department of Biology, Faculty of Science, Genomic Center of Human Pathologies, Faculty of Medicine, Laboratory of Human Pathologies Biology, Mohammed V University, Rabat, Morocco

CHAPTER 1

Biological and Physical Contaminants in Anti-Diabetic Herbal Medicines of Bangladesh

Rausan Zamir[1,*], Nazmul Islam[2,5], Sunzid Ahmed[3], Md. Ali Asraf[1], Nikhil C. Bhoumik[4], Omar Faruque[5] and Akhter Farooque[1]

[1] *Department of Chemistry, University of Rajshahi, Rajshahi, Bangladesh*

[2] *Department of General Educational Development, Daffodil International University, Dhaka, Bangladesh*

[3] *Centre for Advanced Research in Science, University of Dhaka, Dhaka, Bangladesh*

[4] *Wazed Miah Science Research Center, Jahangirnagar University, Savar, Dhaka, Bangladesh*

[5] *Department of Nutrition and Food Technology, Jashore University of Science and Technology, Jashore, Bangladesh*

Abstract: The present study evaluated biological and physical contamination in terms of microbes and toxic metal, respectively, in eight antidiabetic herbal medicines (ADHMs) from different markets in Dhaka City, Bangladesh. Coliform, *E. coli*, *Salmonella* spp. and *Listeria* spp. were absent in all ADHMs. However, aerobic bacterial count of all the samples of yeasts and molds in some samples fails to satisfy safe limits set by different regulatory standards. Among the nine metals [Copper (Cu), Zinc (Zn), Lead (Pb), Manganese (Mn), Chromium (Cr), Iron (Fe), Cadmium (Cd), Nickel (Ni), and Arsenic (As)] investigated, Cu, Zn, Pb, Cr, Ni content was in safe limit according to different pharmacopoeia and WHO guidelines. Among all the regulatory authorities, only the Health Sciences Authority (HSA), Singapore claims the Cd content is above the permissible limit in all the samples except ADHM-4. Chinese pharmacopoeia restricts the use of ADHM-1, ADHM-2 and ADHM-8 because of unacceptable arsenic (As) contamination. All the targeted antidiabetic herbal medicines (ADHMs) were found to retain an unacceptable level of Mn, ranging from 0.44 ± 0.01 to 4.17 ± 0.03 ppm. Metals contamination poses potential risks to human health and regulatory authorities not only should impose a restriction on the use of the medicines but also direct guidelines to keep the drugs safe.

Keywords: ADHMs, Human health and drug safety, Metal toxicity, Microbes.

---

[*] **Corresponding author Rausan Zamir:** Department of Chemistry, University of Rajshahi, Rajshahi, Bangladesh; Tel: +88-01711-705705; Fax: +88-0721-750064; E-mail: rsnzamir@gmail.com

Anna Capasso (Ed.)

INTRODUCTION

Sometimes the conventional medicinal system fails to successfully treat some illnesses [1 - 3]. This inability results in a negative medical encounter, which badly affects the doctor-patient relationship [4 - 6]. As a result, being repulsive with conventional medicine and being attracted to some sort of values and beliefs, also referred to as postmodern philosophy, a fraction of people turns to the alternate medicinal system [4, 7, 8]. In Bangladesh, people are not required to pay extra money to the physician for a prescription and for traditional treatment, no practitioner suggests diagnosis for the investigation disorder related to physic. Therefore, people pay only for traditional drugs. Moreover, the high cost and side effects of most modern drugs shifted consumer's attention from conventional to herbal medicines [9]. Therefore, the uses of herbal medicines are increasing day by day throughout the world [10]. Consumer awareness has increased with the work of ad agencies who are airing undue respectability and credibility of herbal products on television and radio programs [11, 12]. These advertisements aim to attract the different age groups of people with their selective presentation. A child requires healthy growth and development. In his youth, the man requires to cope with daily stress and prevent or slow the onset of aging. While counting his last days on earth, the older one requires to rejuvenate himself. This journey with the requirements mentioned is incomplete without herbal remedies, which supply nutrition and essential ingredients at every step of life to maintain physic [12].

The availability of herbal remedies surpassed drug stores and entered food stores and supermarkets. About 80% of the world's population, living in the developing world, relies on herbal medicinal products as primary healthcare [9, 13, 14]. With this surge of growing use of herbal medicinal products, a whopping number of herbal preparations are incoming and concern related to safety is surging. A notable share of herbal medicine is used as antidiabetic herbal medicine (ADHM)- due to the number of people suffering from diabetes-related complications crossing 200 million worldwide [15, 16].

Metals are widely distributed in nature and occur freely in soil and water. When the metal has a relatively high density and is toxic at low concentration, it is inked as heavy metal. Among the heavy metals, mercury, lead, arsenic and cadmium are toxic metals and have mutagenic effects even at a very low concentration. Mercury was used to treat syphilis before the introduction of penicillin. Another heavy metal, arsenic, is used for the treatment of some forms of malignancy in the compound form [17, 18]. Therefore, the presence of toxic metals as a physical contaminant in herbal remedies is likely. Metal toxicity may lead to malfunction and malformation of organs. Lead poisoning may cause abdominal pain, vomiting, severe anemia, hemoglobulinuria with dark color stools [17, 18].

A wide spectrum of microorganisms has made their adobe in medicinal plants. A series of influences from animal and inanimate sources is behind this hosting. Bacterial endospore and fungal spores are prime microbial loads associated with herbal plants. These varieties of microbial load are transferred to herbal preparations. Intrinsic and extrinsic factors determine the microbial load of medicinal plants. Certain microbial contaminants may cause severe damage to human health. Certain fungal genera produce mycotoxin, which is a potential health hazard chemical. Ingestion of adherent fungal flora with herbal drugs is associated with human disorders. Not only the microbes but also the low molecular weight metabolites from molds are known as chemical contaminants. Improper handling during production and packaging may give access to microbial load to be into herbal drugs. When plastics, glass and other packaging materials come in contact with medicinal herbs, contamination takes place.

While some herbal medicines have proved potential, many of them remain un-assessed in terms of their safety and efficacy [19]. The absence of proper quality controls, improper labeling and inappropriate patient information are behind the compromised quality of herbal drugs [20]. Herbal drugs are introduced as foods or dietary supplements in some countries. By doing so, the quality, efficacy, and safety of these herbal medicines are not required to comply with drug safety regulations. If tested, then quality tests and production standards are less rigorous or controlled. Not only this, the practitioners who are prescribing the health products, may not be certified or licensed. This would leave the safety of the general public on the verge of decaying [21]. The unlicensed herbal remedy is the commonest route which does not have to meet specific standards of safety and quality, neither is it required to be accompanied by safety information for the consumer [20]. Bangladesh is one of the most populous countries, positioning eighth in the world (Fig. **1**). (https://www.infoplease.com/world/population-statistics/worlds-50-most-populous-countries-2016). With small territory, this huge population has made Bangladesh one of the most densely populated in the world.

Unsurprisingly, for a high population with limited wealth, herbal medicines are widely used as medication in Bangladesh. Therefore, the need to educate the physician as well as the general public with adequate information regarding the risks associated with the use of herbal medicines is in demand. With this understanding, a safety investigation of some antidiabetic herbal medicines (ADHMs) in terms of toxic metals (physical contaminants) and microbes (biological contaminants) was taken as our current study.

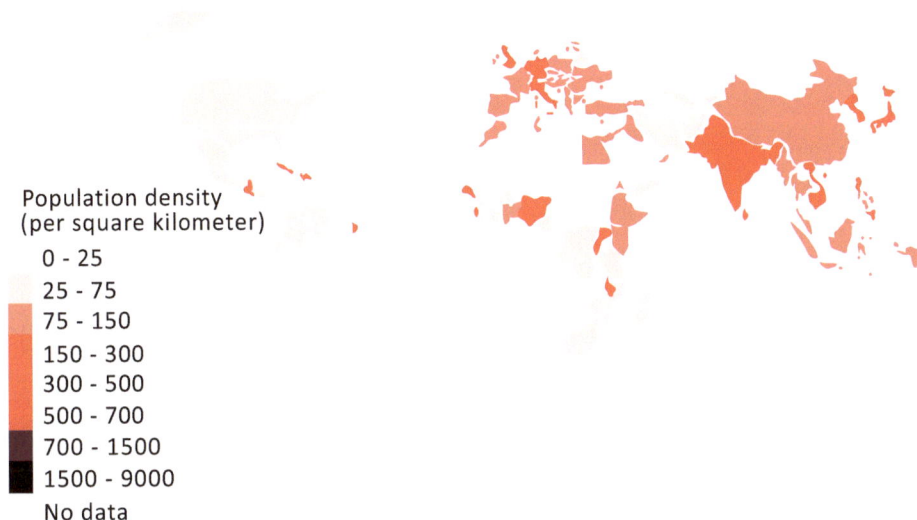

Fig. (1). World Population Distribution.

METHODS

Study Area and Sample Collection

Samples of eight antidiabetic herbal medicines (ADHMs) as finished commercial packs were purchased randomly from different herbal medicine outlets of Dhaka City. Initially, all the samples were prepared for analysis in the research laboratory of Daffodil International University (DIU), Dhaka, Bangladesh. Microbiological contamination and heavy metal content were analyzed in the Center for Advanced Research in Sciences (CARS), University of Dhaka, Bangladesh.

Determination of pH

The pH of different herbal medicines was determined by using a microprocessor pH meter (HI 2210; Hanna Instrument, USA) [17]. For pH determination, the sample solution was prepared by dissolving 12.5 g in 100 mL sterile distilled water with shaking to obtain a homogeneous solution. By means of a microprocessor pH meter, the solution pH of the different herbal medicines was measured and the data were presented as the average of triplicate.

Microbiological Analysis

Preparation of Culture Media

All the media for microbiological analysis were prepared according to the guidelines of manufacturers' and sterilized either in an autoclave (CL-32S; ALP Co. Ltd, Japan) at 121°C and 15 psi pressure for 40 minutes, or by heating in a microwave oven when necessary. The sterile media were dispensed or poured into the sterilized Petri dishes or test tubes as required. The sterility of the prepared media was confirmed by incubating blindly selected plates at 37 °C overnight.

Isolation and Identification of Microorganisms

Isolation of microorganisms was done by following standard surface plate technique on various selective and non-selective agar media. For microbial isolation, samples (25 g, when tablets; 25 mL, when syrup) were homogenized with 225 mL autoclaved normal saline (0.85% NaCl). Same amounts of samples were blended separately into different types of pre-enrichment or enrichment broths (225 mL) in case of presence or absence tests for pathogenic microorganisms.

Total Aerobic Bacterial Count and Total Coliform Count

Sample pH was controlled within the range of 6.9 - 7.9 by adding NaOH or HCl when necessary. For microbial isolation, the samples were serially diluted, and with appropriate dilution, 0.1 mL sample was surface plated on a Tryptic Soy agar (TSA; Oxoid Ltd, Hampshire, England) medium and incubated at 35 °C for 24 hrs. To assess the hygiene of the drug formulations, the total coliform count (TCC) was analyzed by following the surface plating technique with 0.1 mL of the sample (as used for TABC) on MacConkey agar (Oxoid, Hampshire, England) and was incubated at 37°C for 24 hrs. All the samples were separately inoculated into the Tryptic Soya broth (Oxoid, England) as a common enrichment medium and incubated at 37 °C for 24 hrs. The broth culture was then streaked onto a MacConkey agar medium and incubated at 37 °C for 24 hrs. The bacterial growth was monitored for further confirmation of the presence or absence of any coliform bacteria in the samples.

Escherichia coli 0157

All the samples were homogenized in the EC medium and incubated at 35°C for 24 hrs. The enriched cultures were streaked onto a Sorbitol MacConkey agar supplemented with Cefixime and potassium tellurite and incubated at 37°C for 24 hrs. For further confirmation of the identification of presumptive colonies, biochemical tests (IMViC) were performed following the standard procedures.

Escherichia coli

All the samples were homogenized in an Enterobacteria enrichment broth-Mossel pre-enrichment medium and incubated at 35 °C for 24 hrs. 1.0 mL aliquots of pre-enriched cultures were mixed with 9 mL of the double strength EC medium and incubated at 37 °C for 24 hrs. One loop full of the culture was inoculated into a 10 mL 1x EC medium with the Durham fermentation tubes and incubated at 42 °C for 24 hrs. Gas production in the Durham tubes was monitored to confirm the presence or absence of *E. coli* into the 1x EC medium.

Salmonella spp.

All the samples were homogenized independently into the buffered peptone water, followed by incubation at 35 °C for 18-20 hrs. 1.0 mL of pre-enrichment culture was mixed with 9.0 mL of both Hanja Tetrathionate and Rappaport-Vassiliadis broth and incubated for 24 hrs at 35°C and 42 °C, respectively. The culture broths were subsequently streaked onto a Bismuth sulfite agar (BSA; Oxoid, England) and incubated at 37 °C for 24 hrs.

Listeria spp.

Both the tablet and syrup samples were independently supplemented with buffered peptone water and incubated at 30 °C for 4 hrs. 10 mL of broth was then transferred to 90 mL of *Listeria* enrichment broth and the incubation was continued for further 24 hrs at 30 °C. Finally, one loop full of culture broth was streaked onto a PALCAM *Listeria* Selective agar (Oxoid, England), which was supplemented with PALCAM selective supplement, and the inoculated culture medium plates were incubated at 35 °C for 24-48 hrs.

Yeasts and Molds Count (YMC)

Total yeasts and mold analyses were performed by following the surface plating technique on the Saboraud's Dextrose agar (AFC chemical, Bangladesh) with the appropriate dilutions of samples, which were homogenized with sterile normal saline (0.85% NaCl). After 5 days of inoculation at 25° C, the agar plates were observed for the growth of yeasts and molds.

Toxic Metal Analysis

Tablet and capsule samples of antidiabetic herbal medicines (ADHMs) were ground into a fine powder using a mortar and a pestle. Then the powdered samples were digested by taking 3g of each ADHM sample into a separate 100 mL quick fitted round bottom flasks (Pyrex, Germany); 50 mL of 69.5% (w/w) HNO_3 was added to each of the flasks and heated until about 10 mL of each of the solution remained, followed by the addition of 2 mL of 60% $HClO_4$ acid, 10 mL of 69.5% (w/w) HNO_3 and 1mL of 98% (w/w) H_2SO_4. The mixtures were further heated in a fume cupboard until the appearance of white fumes. The resulting solutions after cooling were filtered into separate 100 mL volumetric flasks and then diluted to the mark with de-ionized water [22]. Copper, Zinc, Lead, Manganese, Chromium, Iron, Cadmium, Nickel were atomized by the flame atomic atomizer and analyzed with Atomic Absorption Spectrophotometer (AAS-7000, Shimadzu Corporation, Japan) using the PDA detector. Arsenic was atomized by graphite furnace atomic atomizer. All the standard solutions (1000ppm) with certificates were purchased from Kanto Chemical Co., Japan. The background correction was done by the D2 lamp method. Analyses were made in triplicate. The detection limits of all the elements were determined before sample solutions were analyzed [23]. The method detection limits (MDL) were Cu (0.7 ppb), Zn (0.5 ppb), Pb (0.7 ppb) Mn (0.0.3 ppb), Cr (0.1 ppb), Cd (0.3 ppb) and As (0.5 ppb) (all for aqueous solutions). The optimum analytical range was 0.5 to 5 absorbance units with a coefficient of variation of 0.05-0.40%. The toxic metal content determination was made on a dry weight basis.

RESULTS

Microbial Contamination

None of the herbal drug samples were found to have contaminated with TCC and other pathogenic microorganisms like *E. coli*, *Salmonella* spp., and *Listeria* spp. TABC were reported in the range of 4.15 ± 0.21 to 6.84 ± 0.17 where maximum TABC were in ADHM-1 and minimum TABC were in ADHM-6. Except for ADHM-6 and ADHM-7, all samples were found containing YMC in the range of 3.48 ± 0.00 to 5.31 ± 0.31 (Table 1). Association of low-quality storage facilities can also be responsible for this kind of contamination, which may affect the shelf life of the herbal products.

Metal Toxicity

Investigation of the metal toxicity in eight antidiabetic herbal Medicines (ADHMs) was conducted by determining elemental content of Cu, Zn, Pb, Mn,

Cr, Fe, Cd, Ni and As (Table **2**). All the metals were detected at some levels in all samples.

Table 1. Biological contamination (microbes) in different antidiabetic herbal medicines.

Herbal Drug Type	Code Name of Herbal Drugs	Solution pH	Microbiological Parameters (Log Cfu/Unit)						
			TABC	TCC BE[1]	TCC AE[2]	*E. coli*	*Salmonella* spp.	*Listeria* spp.	YMC
Tablet	ADHM 1	5.3	4.15 ± 0.21	<1.0[4]	A[3]	A	A	A	3.48 ± 0.00
	ADHM 2	5.45	4.59 ± 0.16	<1.0	A	A	A	A	4.23 ± 0.26
	ADHM 3	5.15	5.04 ± 0.24	<1.0	A	A	A	A	4.68 ± 0.06
	ADHM 4	5.55	4.98 ± 0.28	<1.0	A	A	A	A	4.15 ± 0.21
Syrup	ADHM 5	4.38	6.19 ± 0.75	<1.0	A	A	A	A	5.31 ± 0.31
	ADHM 6	6.6	6.84 ± 0.17	<1.0	A	A	A	A	<1.0
	ADHM 7	3.7	4.24 ± 0.34	<1.0	A	A	A	A	<1.0

1= Before enrichment; 2= After enrichment; 3= Absent; 4= Below detection limit (Lowest detection limit is 1.0 log CFU/unit)

Table 2. Physical contaminants (toxic metal) in different antidiabetic herbal medicines.

Code Name of Herbal Drugs	Toxic Metal (Ppm)								
	Cu	Zn	Pb	Mn	Cr	Fe	Cd	Ni	As
ADHM-1	0.11 ±0.02	1.97 ±0.02	0.16 ±0.01	3.44 ±0.03	0.02 ±0.01	0.72 ±0.01	0 ±0.00	0.06 ±0.01	5.22 ±0.02
ADHM-2	0.25 ±0.02	1.73 ±0.02	0.25 ±0.01	4.17 ±0.03	0 ±0.00	10.73 ±0.03	0.02 ±0.01	0.04 ±0.01	6.74 ±0.02
ADHM-3	0.06 ±0.01	0.44 ±0.01	0.15 ±0.01	0.44 ±0.01	0.04 ±0.01	3.74 ±0.02	0 ±0.00	0.04 ±0.01	0.06 ±0.01
ADHM-4	0.09 ±0.01	0.64 ±0.02	0.13 ±0.01	1.33 ±0.02	0.03 ±0.01	4.18 ±0.02	0 ±0.00	0.02 ±0.01	0.65 ±0.01
ADHM-5	0.24 ±0.02	1.51 ±0.03	0.17 ±0.01	0.8 ±0.01	0.01 ±0.01	3.8 ±0.02	0.01 ±0.01	0.03 ±0.01	0.31 ±0.01
ADHM-6	0.46 ±0.02	1.93 ±0.02	0.22 ±0.01	2.34 ±0.02	0.02 ±0.01	4.6 ±0.02	0.01 ±0.01	0.04 ±0.01	0.23 ±0.01

(Table 2) cont.....

ADHM-7	0.05	0.89	0.09	1.26	0.01	7.01	0	0.02	1
	±0.01	±0.01	±0.01	±0.01	±0.01	±0.03	±0.00	±0.01	±0.03
ADHM-8	0.07	1.44	0.17	0.91	0.02	5.4	0.08	0.04	4.34
	±0.01	±0.01	±0.01	±0.02	±0.01	±0.02	±0.01	±0.02	±0.03

Cu was found in the range of 0.05±0.01- 0.46±0.02 ppm in all of the eight ADHMs. The highest and lowest value of Zn was found as 0.44± ppm and 1.97±0.02 ppm in ADHM-3 and ADHM-1, respectively. ADHM-2 was found containing the highest amount of Pb (0.25±0.01 ppm), among eight ADHMs, ADHM-7 was found with the lowest Pb 0.09±ppm. Cd was undetected in ADHM-1, ADHM-3, ADHM-4 and ADHM-7 and its values ranged from 0.08±0.01 ppm in ADHM-8 to 0.01±0.01 ppm in ADHM-2 and ADHM-3, respectively. A considerable amount of As was found in ADHM-1, 2, 7 and 8 as 5.22±0.02 ppm, 6.74±0.02ppm, 1±0.03 ppm and 4.34±0.03 ppm, respectively among eight ADHMs. With the highest and lowest values of 4.17±0.03 ppm in ADHM-2 and 0.44 ppm in ADHM-3, the range of Mn was 0.44±0.01- 4.17±0.3 ppm. The lowest amount of Cr was in ADHM-5 and ADHM-7 among eight ADHMs, with one below detection level valued 0.01±0.01 ppm. The highest amount of Cr was detected in ADHM- 3 (0.03 ppm±0.01). Ni had a range of 0.02±0.01- 0.06±0.01 ppm. The richest Fe containing ADHM was ADHM- 2 with a value of 10.73±0.03 ppm whereas ADHM-1 (0.72±0.01 ppm) was the least Fe containing ADHM.

DISCUSSION

Biological Contamination (Microbes)

The absence of TCC and other pathogenic microorganisms like *E. coli*, *Salmonella* spp., and *Listeria* spp. was reported in all seven ADHM samples. This indicates the raw materials that are prepared from herbal drugs, like leaves or extracts and water were free from fecal or other types of microbial contamination. However, the aerobic bacterial population was found in all the tablet and syrup samples beyond the safe standard range set by the British Pharmacopoeia Commission 2004. The microbiological quality of some samples was also seen as unsatisfactory in terms of unacceptable levels of yeasts and molds contamination. Contact of airborne microbiological contaminants with the drug samples during the production could be the reason for the contamination of herbal drug samples with Y&M and TABC (Table **1**).

Physical Contamination (Metal Toxicity)

Cu was found in the range of 0.05±0.01- 0.46 ±0.02 ppm in all the eight ADHMs. Regulatory bodies like WHO, US FDA, HAS Singapore and Chinese Pharmacopoeia have set their individual specific allowable limit for Cu as 20, 20 150 and 20 ppm, respectively. The ceiling of the range of Cu content 0.46±0.02 ppm in all ADHMs was way below the allowable limits set by the regulatory bodies. Therefore, the medicines were within a safe limit in terms of Cu (Table 3). The permissible limit for Zn is 50 ppm in both WHO and US FDA Guidelines for herbal preparations. The highest value of Zn was found in ADHM-1 as 1.97 is below the permissible limit set by WHO and US FDA of 50 ppm. Hence, Zn is said to have been found within the permissible limit set by regulatory bodies. (Table 3).

Table 3. Permissible limit of heavy metal (ppm) in different antidiabetic herbal medicines.

Toxic Metal	Permissible Limit (Ppm)			
	WHO	US FDA	HSA Singapore	Chinese Pharmacopoeia
Cu	20	20	150	20
Zn	50	50	-	-
Pb	10	10	20	5
Cd	0.2	0.3	0.05	0.3
As	10	10	5	2

The highest value of Pb (0.25±0.01 ppm) was the safe limit set by the WHO (10 ppm) and US FDA (10 ppm). The more lax permissible limit set by HAS Singapore (20 ppm) and stricter permissible limit set by Chinese Pharmacopoeia (5 ppm) also set Pb within the safe limit (Table 3). Cd was found as one of the least appearing metals in all the eight ADHMs where half samples were undetected with Cd (ADHM-1, ADHM-3, ADHM-4 and ADHM-7) with its highest value observed in ADHM-8 as 0.08±0.01ppm. The lowest value of Cd is also the lowest value of all metal content in all the eight ADHMs. Regulatory bodies pose a strict allowable limit for Cd content in ADHMs. The highest Cd containing ADHM, ADHM-8 (0.08±0.01 ppm), was passed to comply with all the regulatory standard body set permissible limits (WHO 0.2 ppm, US FDA 0.3 ppm, Chinese Pharmacopoeia 0.3 ppm) and failed to comply with the HAS Singapore set permissible limit. Therefore, in terms of WHO, US FDA and Chinese Pharmacopoeia, all the ADHMs were within safe limits in terms of Cd. But while considering HAS Singapore, the samples were screened and ADHM-4 was found beyond the safe limit and unsafe (Table 3). Tissue injury is a result of cadmium toxicity [24 - 26]. Tissue injury due to Cadmium toxicity is associated with hypertension, diabetes as cadmium toxicity can lead to insulin resistance [27, 28]. So, while all the ADHMs are used in treating diabetes, the ADHM-4 can escalate the appearance of diabetes. Indeed, it is a shocking result.A relatively higher amount of As is found in ADHM-1, 2, 7 and 8 as 5.22 ± 0.02 ppm, 6.74 ± 0.02ppm, 1 ± 0.03 ppm and 4.34 ± 0.03 ppm, respectively among eight ADHMs. These values of As passes relative relax safe standard by WHO and US FDA (both 10 ppm as a permissible limit for As). However, a strict allowable standard set by HAS Singapore (5 ppm) marks ADHM-2 as unsafe. Moreover, a stricter permissible standard set by Chinese pharmacopoeia (2 ppm) restricts the usage as unsafe in ADHM- 1, ADHM-2 and ADHM-8 (Table **3**).

Mn was found in the range of 0.44 ± 0.01- 4.17 ± 0.03 ppm. The Highest Mn content was found in ADHM- 2 (4.17 ± 0.03 ppm) and the lowest content of Mn was found in ADHM- 3 (0.44 ± 0.01 ppm). The permissible limit for Mn was set at 0.26 ppm [29]. Therefore, all the ADHM samples were failed to comply with safety. Principle toxic effect of Mn is attributed to the effect on the central nervous system (CNS) in the human body [29]. ADHM-5 and ADHM-7were found containing the lowest amount of Cr among eight ADHMs, with one below detection level valued 0.01 ± 0.01 ppm. The Highest amount of Cr was detected in ADHM- 3 (0.04 ± 0.01 ppm). The allowable limit for Cr in herbal preparation is set at 0.05 ppm [29] and this limit is above 0.04 ± 0.01 ppm (ADHM-3 — the highest Cr containing ADHM). Therefore, investigated ADHMs were safe in terms of the Cr content.

Ni was found in the range of 0.02 ± 0.01- 0.06 ± 0.01 ppm. The allowable limit of Ni is 10 ppm (WHO, 1999). All the ADHMs under investigation were found safe as their range (0.02 ± 0.01- 0.06 ± 0.01 ppm) lies below the allowable limit of Ni (10 ppm)ADHM- 2 was richest in Fe with a value of 10.73 ± 0.03 ppm. 0.72 ± 0.01 ppm was the lowest value of Fe in ADHM-1. Oxygen supply, energy production, and immunity in the human body are functioned in the presence of iron, but within the limit. On the contrary, iron overdose leads to dizziness, nausea and vomiting, diarrhea, joints pain, shock, and liver damage. Iron toxicity is attributed to metabolic disorder [30]. The biological and physical contamination results showed that all the samples are recommended unsafe for human consumption due to retaining an unacceptable level of TABC, and Mn content. Apart from this, all the samples except ADHM-6 and ADHM-7 were also found contaminated with the unsatisfactory level of YMC. However, none of the pathogenic microorganisms like *E. coli*, *Salmonella* spp., and *Listeria* spp. was evident in the samples analyzed. However, the presence of aerobic bacterial count in all the samples and YMC also in few samples is drawing attention towards faulty processing and/or storage facilities of bulk raw materials and final. An eye to the processing and manufacturing facility is also suggested figuring out the possible source(s) of TABC and YMC contamination. In essence, from production to storage GMP, GSP should be followed to resist microbial contamination. The samples among nine ADHMs Cu, Zn, Pb Cr, Ni content were not a matter of concern as they have different pharmacopoeia and WHO guidelines. Cd content was found unsafe in Only ADHM-4 of all ADHMs, just according to HAS, Singapore. Arsenic content was above safe range in ADHM-1, ADHM-2 and ADHM-8, only according to Chinese Pharmacopoeia. The microbial and metal contamination in drug samples is always abrupt, which poses potential human health risks. The level and types of microbiological contamination evident may also affect the shelf life of the drug samples. It is advisable that those samples which failed to complying standards with respect to limits set by regulatory bodies in terms of microbial contamination and metal toxicity should not be used. Moreover, there should be a cautious eye over the use of herbal drugs as the efficacy of many products is yet to be proven.

CONSENT FOR PUBLICATION

Not Applicable.

CONFLICT OF INTEREST

The author declares no conflict of interest, financial or otherwise.

ACKNOWLEDGEMENTS

The research work was supported and funded by Swedish International Development Cooperation Agency (SIDA) through International Science Program (ISP), Uppsala University, Sweden.

REFERENCES

[1]   Anyinam C. Alternative medicine in western industrialised countries: and agenda for medical geography. Can Geogr 1990; 34: 69-76.
[http://dx.doi.org/10.1111/j.1541-0064.1990.tb01069.x]

[2]   Lngliss B, West R. The alternative health guide. London: Michael Joseph 1983.

[3]   Holden C. Holistic health concepts gaining momentum. Science 1978; 200(4345): 1029.

[4]   Easthope G. The Response of orthodox medicine to the challenge of alternative medicine in Australia. Aust N Z J Sociol 1993; 29(3): 289-301.
[http://dx.doi.org/10.1177/144078339302900301]

[5]   Sharma UM. Using alternative therapies: marginal medicine and central concerns. In: Abbot P, Payne G, Eds. New Directions in the sociology of health . London: Routledge 1990; p. 13.

[6]   Taylor RCR. Alternative medicine and the medical encounter in Britain and the United States. In: Salmon JW, Ed. Alternative medicines: popular and policy perspectives. New York: Tavistock 1984; pp. 191-228.

[7]   Bakx K. The 'eclipse' of folk medicine in western society. Sociol Health Illn 1991; 13(1): 20-38.

[http://dx.doi.org/10.1111/1467-9566.ep11340307]

[8]   Coward R. The whole truth: the rnyfh ofalternofive medicine. London: Fdber and Faber 1989.

[9]   Bandaranayake WM. Quality control, screening, toxicity, and regulation of herbal drugs. In: Ahmad I, Aqil F, Owais M, Eds. Modern Phytomedicine: Turning Medicinal Plants into Drugs. Germany: Wiley-VCH Verlag GmbH & Co. KGaA 2006; pp. 25-57.

[10]   WHO. WHO Guidelines on Safety Monitoring of Herbal Medicines in Pharmacovigilance Systems. Geneva, Switzerland: World Health Organization 2004.

[11]   Brevort P. The booming us botanical market: a new overview. Herbal Gram 1998; 44: 33-48.

[12]   Parle M, Bansal N. Herbal medicines: are they safe? Nat Prod Radiance 2006; 5: 6-14.

[13]   Mukherjee PW. Quality Control of Herbal Drugs: An Approach to Evaluation of Botanicals. New Delhi, India: Business Horizons Publishers 2002.

[14]   Bodeker C, Bodeker G, Ong CK, Grundy CK, Burford G, Shein K. WHO Global Atlas of Traditional, Complementary and Alternative Medicine. Geneva, Switzerland: World Health Organization 2005.

[15]   Wild S, Roglic G, Green A, Sicree R, King H. Global prevalence of diabetes: estimates for the year 2000 and projections for 2030. Diabetes Care 2004; 27(5): 1047-53.
        [http://dx.doi.org/10.2337/diacare.27.5.1047] [PMID: 15111519]

[16]   McCune LM, Johns T. Antioxidant activity in medicinal plants associated with the symptoms of diabetes mellitus used by the indigenous peoples of the North American boreal forest. J Ethnopharmacol 2002; 82(2-3): 197-205.
        [http://dx.doi.org/10.1016/S0378-8741(02)00180-0] [PMID: 12241996]

[17]   Gogtay NJ, Bhatt HA, Dalvi SS, Kshirsagar NA. The use and safety of non-allopathic Indian medicines. Drug Saf 2002; 25(14): 1005-19.
        [http://dx.doi.org/10.2165/00002018-200225140-00003] [PMID: 12408732]

[18]   Ernst E, Thompson Coon J. Heavy metals in traditional Chinese medicines: a systematic review. Clin Pharmacol Ther 2001; 70(6): 497-504.
        [http://dx.doi.org/10.1067/mcp.2001.120249] [PMID: 11753265]

[19]   WHO. Traditional Medicine Strategy (2002–2005) WHO/EDM/TRM/20021. Geneva, Switzerland: World Health Organization 2002. b

[20]   Raynor DK, Dickinson R, Knapp P, Long AF, Nicolson DJ. Buyer beware? Does the information provided with herbal products available over the counter enable safe use? BMC Med 2011; 9: 94.
        [http://dx.doi.org/10.1186/1741-7015-9-94] [PMID: 21827684]

[21]   Kasilo OMJ, Trapsida JM. Decade of African traditional medicine, 2001–2010. Afr Health Monit 2011; 14: 25-31.

[22]   Miller-Ihli JN, Baker AS. Food and dairy products, applications of atomic spectroscopy encyclopedia of spectroscopy and spectrometry. London: Academic press 2000; Vol. 1: pp. 583-8.

[23]   Varian Techtron. Basic Atomic Absorption Spectroscopy – A Modern Introduction. Springvale, Australia: Varian Techtron 1975; pp. 104-6.

[24]   Matrovic V, Buha A, Bulat Z. Cadmium toxicity revisited: focus on oxidative stress induction and interactions with zinc and magnesium. Arhiv za Higijenu Rada i Toksikologiju 2011; 62(1): 65-76.

[25]   Patra RC, Rautray AK, Swarup D. Oxidative stress in lead and cadmium toxicity and its amelioration. Vet Med Int 2011; 2011: 457327.

[26]   Cuypers A, Plusquin M, Remans T, *et al*. Cadmium stress: an oxidative challenge. Biometals 2010; 23(5): 927-40.
        [http://dx.doi.org/10.1007/s10534-010-9329-x] [PMID: 20361350]

[27]   Satarug S, Moore MR. Emerging roles of cadmium and heme oxygenase in type-2 diabetes and cancer

susceptibility. Tohoku J Exp Med 2012; 228(4): 267-88.
[http://dx.doi.org/10.1620/tjem.228.267] [PMID: 23117262]

[28]   Chen YW, Yang CY, Huang CF, Hung DZ, Leung YM, Liu SH. Heavy metals, islet function and diabetes development. Islets 2009; 1(3): 169-76.
[http://dx.doi.org/10.4161/isl.1.3.9262] [PMID: 21099269]

[29]   Sathiavelu A, Gajalakshmi S, Iswarya V, Ashwini R, Divya G, Mythili S. Evaluation of heavy metals in medicinal plants growing in Vellore District. Eur J Exp Biol 2012; 2(5): 1457-61.

[30]   Martin S, Griswold W. Human health effects of heavy metals, Environmental Science and Technology briefs for citizens, Centre for Hazardous Substance Research. 2009; 15: pp. 1-6.

CHAPTER 2

Quantification and Health Safety Assessment of Some Toxic Metals in Anti-Diabetic Herbal Preparations Collected from Local Retailers Using the XRF Analytical Tool

Rausan Zamir[1,*], Nazmul Islam[2,4], Mahfuza Parveen[3], Shipra Sarker[4], Rajib Kanti[4], M. Safiur Rahman[5] and Omar Faruque[4]

[1] *Department of Chemistry, University of Rajshahi, Rajshahi, Bangladesh*

[2] *Department of General Educational Development, Daffodil International University, Dhaka, Bangladesh*

[3] *Department of Environmental Science and Disaster Management, Daffodil International University, Dhaka-1207, Bangladesh*

[4] *Department of Nutrition and Food Technology, Jashore University of Science and Technology, Jashore, Bangladesh*

[5] *Atmospheric and Environmental Chemistry Laboratory, Chemistry Division, Atomic Energy Center, 4-Kazi Nazrul Islam Avenue, Dhaka-1000, Bangladesh*

Abstract: In developing countries, an increase of diabetes became an alarming issue and recognized as the third leading fatal disorder among all syndromes. Bangladesh also has a large number of diabetic people in the world. In the present study, the quantification of major toxic metals and the assessment of their safety in the anti-diabetic herbal preparations had been undertaken. In our investigation, a handful of samples collected randomly from different kiosks and herbal retail shops in Dhaka city, Bangladesh, were exposed to the X-ray fluorescence (XRF) technique. It was found that the average concentration of calcium was the highest (660.82mg/50gm) and arsenic was the lowest in concentrations (<0.01mg/50gm) in all anti-diabetic herbal preparations (ADHPs). Cu, Fe and Ni concentration above the safety limits and two samples containing Zn concentration above the safety limits were recommended by WHO and FAO as 3 ppm, 20 ppm, 1.63 ppm and 50 ppm for herbal drugs, respectively. Other toxic heavy metals like As, Pb and Co were found with a respective concentration of <0.01, <0.012 and <0.22 mg/50 gm, which were all within their safe consumption limit. Patients who take the herbal drugs can suffer from dizziness, nausea and vomiting, dermatitis, irritation of the upper respiratory tract, abdominal pain, diarrhea, joints pain, shock, and even liver damage due to the overdose of iron and zinc.

---

* **Corresponding author Rausan Zamir:** Department of Chemistry, University of Rajshahi, Rajshahi, Bangladesh; Tel: +88-01711-705705; Fax: +88-0721-750064; E-mail: rsnzamir@gmail.com

Based on the present study, it can be clarified that the percentage of heavy metal concentrations in herbal drugs in Bangladesh is at risk. Regulatory agencies should come forward and take the necessary measures to ensure the safety of finished herbal preparations.

Keywords: Anti-diabetic herbal preparations (ADHP), Heavy metal, X-ray fluorescence (XRF).

INTRODUCTION

Numerous diseases [1] are cured by herbal remedies due to the presence of active pharmacological components [2] in them. Eighty percent of people in the developing countries rely on herbal medicines as their primary healthcare [3, 4], and about 25% of the drugs prescribed worldwide are plant derived [5]. By 2030, 90% cases will be attributed to type-2 diabetes and their complications will reach 552 million people [6], which will be 7% of the world population. And by 2035, the number of patients from diabetes will constitute a 10% population of the world, which will be 592 million people [7, 8]. Therapeutic efficacy of relatively low cost in comparison with other medications and low side effects [9, 10] is gaining attention as ailment of diabetes type-2. Herbal formulations are inherently safe, as they are originated naturally. However, toxicity and adverse effects are not uncommon [11]. Contaminants such as pesticides, microbes, heavy metals, chemical toxins, and adulterants are held responsible for the toxicity of herbal remedies [12]. Both natural and anthropogenic sources, like the geochemical characteristics of soil and contaminants in the soil, water, and air, and others during growth, transport, and storage conditions, make a passage for the contaminants. The use of heavy metals [13, 14] in herbal formulations can have a synergistic effect [15] and amplify drug efficacy. Heavy metal, like Ni, plays an important role in insulin production [16], however, exerts a potent toxic effect on peripheral tissues and on the reproductive system [17]. For proper insulin functioning, the human body requires Mn [18]. Therefore, there is a possibility of intentional adulteration of ADHPs with Mn in the management of diabetes. Recently, toxicity due to trace metals has gained considerable attention considering their impact on human health [19 - 28].

While analyzing a sample in terms of heavy metal, the destruction of the sample bulk matrix takes place during sample preparation in popular analytical tools like ICP and AAS. However, XRF allows non-destructive analysis [29], ensuring reliability, precision and sensitivity of results when there exists a small range between deficiency and toxicity for the human body of metals. Quantification and health safety assessment of some toxic metals in anti-diabetic herbal preparations using the XRF analytical tool has been taken as a research objective.

METHODS

Study Area and Sample Collection

Anti-diabetic herbal preparation (ADHPs) is a finished commercial pack with different brands randomly collected from different kiosks and herbal retail shops of Dhaka City, Bangladesh (Table 1). Medicines were collected in airtight plastic containers or glass bottles depending on their physical state, followed by the date of manufacturing, date of expiring and batch numbers tabulating.

Sample Preparation and Analysis

Oven-dried (35^0C for 5 minutes) samples were pulverized to a fine powder and pressed into a pellet of 13 mm size using a CARVER model manual pelletizer (6-8ton pressure). Samples were bombarded by the x-ray tube (25 V, 50 Micro A for 100 counts) and detected by a solid-state Si- Li detector. Through ADMCA and FP-CROSS software, the spectrum was analyzed. Results and figures were summarized using Microsoft Excel 2013.

Table 1. Anti-diabetic herbal preparations under investigation (n=22).

SL No	Code	Dosage Form	Dosage	Weight per Tablet or Capsule (MG)	SL No	Code	Dosage Form	Dosage	Weight per Tablet or Capsule (MG)
1	ADHP-01	Tablet	1-3 tab, 2-3 times	665	12	ADHP-12	Capsule	1 capsule, 2-3 times	505
2	ADHP-02	Capsule	1-2 capsule, 1-2 times	620	13	ADHP-13	Tablet	1-2 tablet, 2-3 times	500
3	ADHP-03	Capsule	2 capsule, 2 times	500	14	ADHP-14	Tablet	1-2 tablet, 2 times	560
4	ADHP-04	Capsule	1 capsule, 3 times	510	15	ADHP-15	Tablet	10 gms, 2-3 times	450
5	ADHP-05	Tablet	1 tablet, 2 times	500	16	ADHP-16	Tablet	2 tablets, 3 times	480
6	ADHP-06	Capsule	1-2 capsule, 1-2 times	500	17	ADHP-17	Tablet	1-2 tablets, 2 times	550
7	ADHP-07	Capsule	1 capsule, 2-3 times	450	18	ADHP-18	Tablet	1-2 tablets, 3 times	3000
8	ADHP-08	Tablet	1 tablet, 2 times	200	19	ADHP-19	Tablet	1-2 tablets, 3 times	690

(Table 1) cont.....

SL No	Code	Dosage Form	Dosage	Weight per Tablet or Capsule (MG)	SL No	Code	Dosage Form	Dosage	Weight per Tablet or Capsule (MG)
9	ADHP-09	Capsule	1 capsule, 2 times	490	20	ADHP-20	Tablet	1 tablet, 1-2 times	550
10	ADHP-10	Tablet	1-2 tablet, 3 times	650	21	ADHP-21	Capsule	1 capsule, 2 times	520
11	ADHP-11	Capsule	1-2 capsule, 2 times	510	22	ADHP-22	Capsule	1-3 capsule, 2 times	480

RESULTS AND DISCUSSION

K content varied between 41.71 mg/50gm (ADHP- 8)- 218.79 mg/50gm (ADHP-3) (Table **2**). The presence of K ion is evident in a wide variety of proteins and enzymes in the human body [30]. Four ADHPs were found with an average calcium concentration as high as 1.5gm/50gm, which can be equivalent to 175mg daily consumption of this mineral. It has been suggested that doses up to 1500 mg/day of supplemental calcium would not expect to result in adverse effects, however, higher doses could result in adverse gastrointestinal symptoms [31].

Table 2. Metal concentration in anti-diabetic herbal preparations (n=22).

SL No	Code	Metal Concentration (Mg/ 50 Gm)											
		K	Ca	Mn	Ni	Co	Cu	Zn	As	Pb	Fe	Rb	Sr
1	ADHP- 01	186.5	415.2	4.6	<0.19	<0.22	0.36	0.49	<0.01	<0.12	13.4	0.86	0.57
2	ADHP- 02	163.8	**2168**	3.6	<0.19	<0.22	0.37	0.4	<0.01	<0.12	20.4	0.84	1.38
3	ADHP- 03	**218.8**	1357.5	12.4	<0.19	<0.22	**0.33**	0.33	<0.01	<0.12	28.2	0.41	1.34
4	ADHP- 04	148.9	484.1	4.2	<0.19	<0.22	0.57	0.48	<0.01	<0.12	20.8	**1.71**	0.71
5	ADHP- 05	57.5	532.5	10.7	<0.19	<0.22	0.8	**10.84**	<0.01	<0.12	**180.7**	1.18	0.97
6	ADHP- 06	161.7	286.5	6.2	<0.19	<0.22	0.35	0.41	<0.01	<0.12	24.5	1.51	0.78
7	ADHP- 07	198.5	396.9	8.2	<0.19	<0.22	0.47	0.42	<0.01	<0.12	14.9	1.93	**2**
8	ADHP- 08	41.7	262.2	3.6	<0.19	<0.22	0.43	0.37	<0.01	<0.12	12.4	0.37	1.31
9	ADHP- 09	149.7	389.1	8	<0.19	<0.22	0.44	0.55	<0.01	<0.12	16.7	1.62	0.82
10	ADHP- 10	70.2	483.4	5.5	<0.19	<0.22	0.52	0.39	<0.01	<0.12	14.6	**0.22**	0.36
11	ADHP- 11	107.2	529.5	7	<0.19	<0.22	0.43	0.33	<0.01	<0.12	128.3	0.67	1.52
12	ADHP- 12	175.4	460.9	4.3	<0.19	<0.22	0.56	0.47	<0.01	<0.12	29.4	1.14	1.47
13	ADHP- 13	**45.6**	1239.5	3.6	<0.19	<0.22	0.36	0.29	<0.01	<0.12	12.8	0.17	0.37
14	ADHP- 14	98.8	1938.5	6.2	<0.19	<0.22	**0.98**	9.07	<0.01	<0.12	83.5	0.67	0.57

(Table 2) cont.....

SL No	Code	Metal Concentration (Mg/ 50 Gm)											
		K	**Ca**	**Mn**	**Ni**	**Co**	**Cu**	**Zn**	**As**	**Pb**	**Fe**	**Rb**	**Sr**
15	ADHP- 15	138.4	**96.5**	**3.5**	<0.19	<0.22	0.41	0.48	<0.01	<0.12	**6.4**	0.39	**0.14**
16	ADHP- 16	78.7	579	**18.5**	<0.19	<0.22	0.63	1.05	<0.01	<0.12	45.5	0.98	0.97
17	ADHP- 17	71.6	796.5	3.7	<0.19	<0.22	0.39	0.38	<0.01	<0.12	11.3	0.39	0.78
18	ADHP- 18	76.6	345.5	4.2	<0.19	<0.22	0.37	0.32	<0.01	<0.12	16.5	1.07	0.29
19	ADHP- 19	51.1	426.6	4.9	<0.19	<0.22	0.39	**0.25**	<0.01	<0.12	10.8	0.67	0.36
20	ADHP- 20	53,9	433.7	5	<0.19	<0.22	0.4	**0.25**	<0.01	<0.12	10.9	0.66	0.36
21	ADHP- 21	176.4	474.8	9	<0.19	<0.22	0.39	0.69	<0.01	<0.12	15.7	1.48	0.64
22	ADHP- 22	146.9	441.6	8.4	<0.19	<0.22	0.46	0.65	<0.01	<0.12	15.2	1.3	1.04

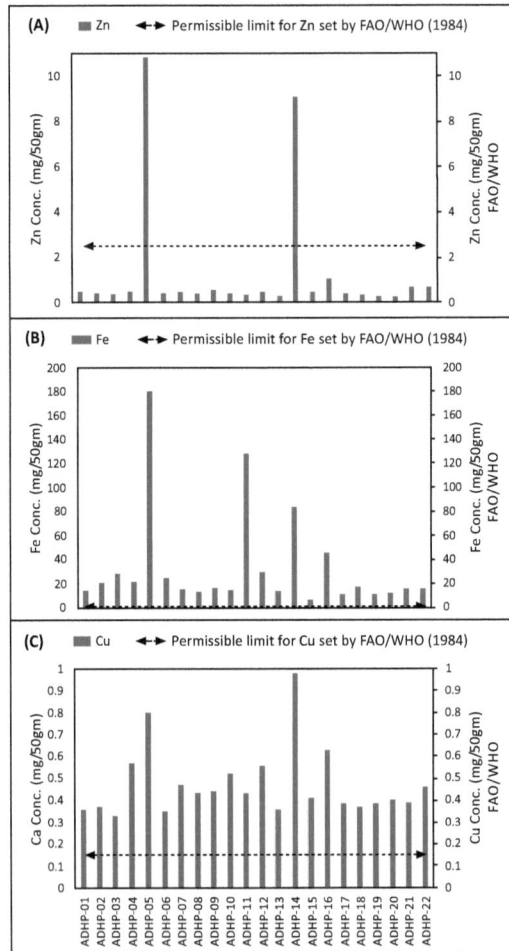

Fig. (1). Health Risk assessment of Zinc, Iron and Copper with respect to **39**.

Only ADHP-16 crossed the permissible limit of daily exposure for Mn. Mn is essential for the normal development of all mammals [32]. However, overexposure to the metal can lead to neurodegenerative damage [33 - 35]. Co content was below 22 mg/50 gm. Thyroid metabolism is assisted by Co. However, a high dose is associated with damaged thyroid [36]. All of the samples contained high levels of Cu crossing the permissible safe limit by WHO/FAO (0.15mg/50gm) (Fig. 1). Prolong exposure can lead to dermatitis, irritation of the upper respiratory tract, abdominal pain, nausea, diarrhea, vomiting, and liver damage [37, 38].

The amount of Zn in the analyzed samples ranged from 0.25 (ADHP 19, ADHP-20) 10.84 (ADHP-5) mg/50 gm (Table **2**). Maximum 2.5 mg/50 gm Zn can be considered safe to uptake (WHO/FAO) which, except ADHP-5 (10.84mg/ 50 gm) and ADHP-14 (9.07 mg/ 50 gm), implies 20 ADHPs were safe to consume. For proper thyroid function, zinc is an essential element required in trace quantity. But if zinc uptake exceeds high zinc permissible limits, it produces toxic effects on the immune system [39]. The Fe concentration varied in a wide range, 6.4 (ADHP-5--180.7 (ADHP- 15) mg/50gm (Table **2**). The concentration of Fe in all ADHPs (6.4mg/50gm or above) crossed the permissible limit (Fig. **1**). The proper functioning of the human body depends on iron; at overdose, organ damage takes place [37]. The presence of Ni was below 0.19 mg/50 gm in all ADHPs (Table **2**). Following the stringent limit of WHO/FAO, the permissibility limit of exposure of Ni (0.08mg/ 50gm) for all ADHPs (0.19mg/50gm) exceeded, which is alarming as Ni is a highly toxic environmental pollutant and the most common metal allergen where 20-40% of female and 3-5% of the male population has Ni allergy contact rate [40]. The maximum permissible level of As in herbal preparations is 0.5mg/50gm recommended by WHO and FAO, indicating all the herbal drugs safe to consume from As toxicity [41, 42]. A meager quantity of Pb (< 0.12mg/50gm) is estimated in all herbal drug samples (Table **2**), implying all the herbal medicines safe from adversity [43] under the permissible limit of exposure (permissible limit: 0.5 mg/ 50 gm). Rb was found between 0.22 (ADHP-10)-1.71 (ADHP-4) mg/50 gm (Table **2**). After entering the human body, Rb^+ ions mimic K^+ ions, and concentrate in the body's intracellular fluid [44]. The ions toxicity is not alarming as a 70 kg person contains average 360 mg of rubidium, which does not affect the individual by increasing Rb concentration 50 to 100 times [45]. Sr was found in the range of 0.14 (ADHP-15)-2 (ADHP-7) mg/50 gm (Table **2**). The average human can intake 2mg/day Sr without harm and its chemical similarity to Ca enables its stable isotopes not to pose a significant health threat [46]. There are a number of factors contributing to heavy metal contamination (agricultural soils, including fertilizers, pesticides, atmospheric deposition from town wastes, industrial emissions [47]). Metal content varied depending on the country of origin, environmental pollution levels, plant part, and processing methods [48,

49]. The health risk due to metal contamination, in general, depends on the average daily intake of these herbal formulations.

CONCLUSION

All samples for metals like Cu, Zn and Fe and two samples for metals such as Zn and Mn crossed their respective permissible safe limit recommended by WHO/FAO. Prolong uptake of these drugs containing these metals may cause toxicity to human health at a certain level. This is very concerning for drug safety and, in turn, would affect public health safety as well. There is a need to implement a regular monitoring and assessment procedure on the quality of local herbal medicines formulated in Bangladesh, which necessitates the establishment of a scientific screening protocol.

CONSENT FOR PUBLICATION

Not Applicable.

CONFLICT OF INTEREST

The author declares no conflict of interest, financial or otherwise.

ACKNOWLEDGEMENTS

Swedish International Development Cooperation Agency (SIDA) aided this research work financially through International Science Program (ISP), Uppsala University, Sweden.

REFERENCES

[1]   Sakkir S, Kabshawi M, Mehairbi M. Medicinal plants diversity and their conservation status in the United Arab Emirates (UAE). J Med Plants Res 2012; 6(7): 1304-22.

[2]   Fabricant DS, Farnsworth NR. The value of plants used in traditional medicine for drug discovery. Environ Health Perspect 2001; 109 (Suppl. 1): 69-75.
[PMID: 11250806]

[3]   Organization WH. Global Tuberculosis Control: Surveillance, Planning, Financing: WHO Report 2008. World Health Organization 2008; Vol. 393.

[4]   Calixto JB. Twenty-five years of research on medicinal plants in Latin America: a personal view. J Ethnopharmacol 2005; 100(1-2): 131-4.
[http://dx.doi.org/10.1016/j.jep.2005.06.004] [PMID: 16006081]

[5]   Rates SMK. Plants as source of drugs. Toxicon 2001; 39(5): 603-13.
[http://dx.doi.org/10.1016/S0041-0101(00)00154-9] [PMID: 11072038]

[6]   Whiting DR, Guariguata L, Weil C, Shaw J. IDF diabetes atlas: global estimates of the prevalence of diabetes for 2011 and 2030. Diabetes Res Clin Pract 2011; 94(3): 311-21.
[http://dx.doi.org/10.1016/j.diabres.2011.10.029] [PMID: 22079683]

[7]   Chen L, Magliano DJ, Zimmet PZ. The worldwide epidemiology of type 2 diabetes mellitus--present

and future perspectives. Nat Rev Endocrinol 2011; 8(4): 228-36.
[http://dx.doi.org/10.1038/nrendo.2011.183] [PMID: 22064493]

[8] Shaw JE, Sicree RA, Zimmet PZ. Global estimates of the prevalence of diabetes for 2010 and 2030. Diabetes Res Clin Pract 2010; 87(1): 4-14.
[http://dx.doi.org/10.1016/j.diabres.2009.10.007] [PMID: 19896746]

[9] Hoareau L, DaSilva EJ. Medicinal plants: a re-emerging health aid. Electron J Biotechnol 1999; 2(2): 3-4.

[10] Iwu MW, Duncan AR, Okunji CO. New antimicrobials of plant. In: Janick J, Ed. Perspectives on new crops and new uses. Alexandria, VA: ASHS Press 1999; pp. 457-62.

[11] Ernst E. Toxic heavy metals and undeclared drugs in Asian herbal medicines. Trends Pharmacol Sci 2002; 23(3): 136-9.
[http://dx.doi.org/10.1016/S0165-6147(00)01972-6] [PMID: 11879681]

[12] Saad B, Azaizeh H, Abu-Hijleh G, Said O. Safety of traditional arab herbal medicine. Evid Based Complement Alternat Med 2006; 3(4): 433-9.
[http://dx.doi.org/10.1093/ecam/nel058] [PMID: 17173106]

[13] Organization WH. Hazardous Chemicals in Human and Environmental Health: A Resource Book for School, College and University Students. Geneva: World Health Organization 2000.

[14] Debas HT, Laxminarayan R, Straus SE. Complementary and Alternative Medicine. In: Jamison DT, Breman JG, Measham AR, Eds. Disease Control Priorities in Developing Countries. 2nd edition., Washington (DC): The International Bank for Reconstruction and Development/The World Bank 2006.

[15] Cindrić IJ, Zeiner M, Glamuzina E, Stingeder G. Elemental characterisation of the medical herbs *Salvia officinalis* L. and *Teucrium montanum* L. grown in Croatia. Microchem J 2013; 107: 185-9.
[http://dx.doi.org/10.1016/j.microc.2012.06.013]

[16] Kabata-Pendias PH. Trace Elements in Soil and Plants. Ann Arbor, London: CRC Pres, Boca Raton 1992.

[17] McGrath SP. Chromium and nickel In: Alloway BJ, Ed. Heavy Met soils. London: Blackie & Sons 1990; pp. 125-50.

[18] Kazi TG, Afridi HI, Kazi N, *et al.* Copper, chromium, manganese, iron, nickel, and zinc levels in biological samples of diabetes mellitus patients. Biol Trace Elem Res 2008; 122(1): 1-18.
[http://dx.doi.org/10.1007/s12011-007-8062-y] [PMID: 18193174]

[19] Rahimi M, Farhadi R, Balashahri MS. Effects of heavy metals on the medicinal plant. Int J Agron Plant Prod 2012; 3(4): 154-8.

[20] Saper RB, Kales SN, Paquin J, *et al.* Heavy metal content of ayurvedic herbal medicine products. JAMA 2004; 292(23): 2868-73.
[http://dx.doi.org/10.1001/jama.292.23.2868] [PMID: 15598918]

[21] Saeed M, Muhammad N, Khan H. Assessment of heavy metal content of branded Pakistani herbal products. Trop J Pharm Res 2011; 10(4): 499-506.
[http://dx.doi.org/10.4314/tjpr.v10i4.16]

[22] Harris ESJ, Cao S, Littlefield BA, *et al.* Heavy metal and pesticide content in commonly prescribed individual raw Chinese Herbal Medicines. Sci Total Environ 2011; 409(20): 4297-305.
[http://dx.doi.org/10.1016/j.scitotenv.2011.07.032] [PMID: 21824641]

[23] Alwakeel SS. Microbial and heavy metals contamination of herbal medicines. Res J Microbiol 2008; 3(12): 683-91.
[http://dx.doi.org/10.3923/jm.2008.683.691]

[24] Mahan LK, Escott-Stump S, Raymond JL, Krause MV. Krause's Food & the Nutrition Care Process. Elsevier Health Sciences 2012.

[25]   Singh R, Gautam N, Mishra A, Gupta R. Heavy metals and living systems: An overview. Indian J Pharmacol 2011; 43(3): 246-53.
        [http://dx.doi.org/10.4103/0253-7613.81505] [PMID: 21713085]

[26]   Centeno JA, Tchounwou PB, Patlolla AK, *et al.* Environmental pathology and health effects of arsenic poisoning. Manag Arsen Environ From Soil to Hum Heal 2006; pp. 311-27.

[27]   Charcot JM. Clinical Lectures on Certain Diseases of the Nervous System. Davis 1888.

[28]   Korfali SI, Hawi T, Mroueh M. Evaluation of heavy metals content in dietary supplements in Lebanon. Chem Cent J 2013; 7(1): 10.
        [http://dx.doi.org/10.1186/1752-153X-7-10] [PMID: 23331553]

[29]   Potts PJ, Ellis AT, Kregsamer P, *et al.* Atomic spectrometry update. X-ray fluorescence spectrometry. J Anal At Spectrom 2005; 20(10): 1124-54.
        [http://dx.doi.org/10.1039/b511542f]

[30]   Vašák M, Schnabl J. Sodium and potassium ions in proteins and enzyme catalysis. In: Sigel A, Sigel H, Sigel R, Eds. The Alkali Metal Ions: Their Role for Life Metal Ions in Life Sciences. Switzerland: Springer, Cham 2016; Vol. 16: pp. 259-90.
        [http://dx.doi.org/10.1007/978-3-319-21756-7_8]

[31]   EGVM Report on safe upper levels for vitamins and minerals. 2003.

[32]   Keen CL, Bell JG, Lönnerdal B. The effect of age on manganese uptake and retention from milk and infant formulas in rats. J Nutr 1986; 116(3): 395-402.
        [http://dx.doi.org/10.1093/jn/116.3.395] [PMID: 3950766]

[33]   Barbeau A. Manganese and extrapyramidal disorders (a critical review and tribute to Dr. George C. Cotzias). Neurotoxicology 1984; 5(1): 13-35.
        [PMID: 6538948]

[34]   Mena I, Marin O, Fuenzalida S, Cotzias GC. Chronic manganese poisoning: Clinical picture and manganese turnover. Neurology 1967; 17(2): 128-36.
        [http://dx.doi.org/10.1212/WNL.17.2.128] [PMID: 6066873]

[35]   Inoue N, Makita Y. Neurological aspects in human exposures to manganese. In: Chang LW, Ed. Toxicology of Metals. Boca Raton, FL: CRC Press 1996; pp. 415-21.

[36]   Bethesda MD US Department of Health and Human Services. National Library of Medicine 1993.

[37]   Martin S, Griswold W. Human health effects of heavy metals. Environ Sci Technol briefs citizens 2009; 15: 1-6.

[38]   Ullah R, Khader JA, Hussain I, Talha NMA, Khan N. Investigation of macro and micro-nutrients in selected medicinal plants. Afr J Pharm Pharmacol 2012; 6(25): 1829-32.

[39]   Fosmire GJ. Zinc toxicity. Am J Clin Nutr 1990; 51(2): 225-7.
        [http://dx.doi.org/10.1093/ajcn/51.2.225] [PMID: 2407097]

[40]   Mathelier-Fusade P, Vermeulen C, Leynadier F. [Vibratory angioedema]. Ann Dermatol Venereol 2001; 128(6-7): 750-2.
        [PMID: 11460039]

[41]   Franzblau A, Lilis R. Acute arsenic intoxication from environmental arsenic exposure. Arch Environ Health 1989; 44(6): 385-90.
        [http://dx.doi.org/10.1080/00039896.1989.9935912] [PMID: 2610527]

[42]   Ng JC, Wang J, Shraim A. A global health problem caused by arsenic from natural sources. Chemosphere 2003; 52(9): 1353-9.
        [http://dx.doi.org/10.1016/S0045-6535(03)00470-3] [PMID: 12867164]

[43]   García-Lestón J, Méndez J, Pásaro E, Laffon B. Genotoxic effects of lead: an updated review. Environ Int 2010; 36(6): 623-36.

[http://dx.doi.org/10.1016/j.envint.2010.04.011] [PMID: 20466424]

[44] Relman AS. The physiological behavior of rubidium and cesium in relation to that of potassium. Yale J Biol Med 1956; 29(3): 248-62.
[PMID: 13409924]

[45] Fieve RR, Meltzer HL, Taylor RM. Rubidium chloride ingestion by volunteer subjects: initial experience. Psychopharmacology (Berl) 1971; 20(4): 307-14.
[http://dx.doi.org/10.1007/BF00403562] [PMID: 5561654]

[46] Emsley J. Nature's Building Blocks: An AZ Guide to the Elements. Oxford University Press 2011.

[47] Garrett RG. Natural sources of metals to the environment. Hum Ecol Risk Assess 2000; 6(6): 945-63.
[http://dx.doi.org/10.1080/10807030091124383]

[48] Chizzola R, Lukas B. Variability of the cadmium content in hypericumSpecies collected in eastern austria. Water Air Soil Pollut 2006; 170(1-4): 331-43.
[http://dx.doi.org/10.1007/s11270-005-9004-y]

[49] Abou-Arab AAK, Abou Donia MA. Heavy metals in Egyptian spices and medicinal plants and the effect of processing on their levels. J Agric Food Chem 2000; 48(6): 2300-4.
[http://dx.doi.org/10.1021/jf990508p] [PMID: 10888541]

CHAPTER 3

Caffeine Intake and the Risk of Female Primary Infertility: An Evidence-Based Case Report

A. Zaifar[1], E.N. Nabila[1], L.D. Vincent[1], N.M.P Kusuma[1], S.S.K. Nareswari[2] and M. Louisa[2,*]

[1] *Faculty of Medicine, Universitas Indonesia, Jakarta, Indonesia*

[2] *Department of Pharmacology and Therapeutics, Faculty of Medicine, Universitas Indonesia, Jakarta, Indonesia*

Abstract: Female primary infertility is a major global challenge known to be influenced by dietary factors, including caffeine intake. Moderate caffeine intake has been proposed to have beneficial health effects while excessive caffeine intake may represent health risks, with the reproductive system being one of them. However, studies regarding the association between high caffeine intake and reduced female infertility are still inconclusive. This evidence-based case report was investigated to know whether daily high caffeine consumption is associated with female primary infertility indicated by time to pregnancy (TTP) and spontaneous abortion (SAB).

A structured literature search for cohort, case-control and meta-analysis was performed using Pubmed and Scopus database. Selected articles were appraised using appraisal tools from CEBM for meta-analysis, and NOS assessment tool for cohort and case-control studies.

Four articles (one meta-analysis, two cohort studies, and one case-control study) were selected based on predefined selection criteria. High caffeine intake was not associated with 12 months TTP based on all studies, except for one case-control study. Whereas, based on the meta-analysis of 27 studies that provided sufficient data on SAB, it was shown that increased caffeine consumption significantly increased the risk of SAB. However, studies that assessed SAB had significant heterogeneity.

In conclusion, based on studies with the highest evidence level and appropriate NOS and CEBM scores, we found an insignificant association, if any, between high caffeine intake and primary infertility based on two indicators, which were TTP and SAB. Therefore, we recommend that women trying to achieve pregnancy do not necessarily need to restrict their caffeine intake.

* **Corresponding author M. Louisa:** Department of Pharmacology and Therapeutics, Faculty of Medicine, Universitas Indonesia, Jakarta, Indonesia; Tel: +62-21-31930481; E-mail: melva.louisa@gmail.com

Keywords: Female primary infertility, High caffeine intake, Spontaneous abortion, Time to pregnancy.

CASE

A couple comes to a fertility clinic with a complaint of inability to conceive after 1 year of actively trying to become pregnant. The husband, 34 years old, is known to have 2 children from his late wife and tested normal for semen variables. The wife, 29 years old, is reported to have no secondary conditions affecting her reproductive system, however, it is reported that she had a spontaneous abortion a year before (gestational age= 7 weeks). During anamnesis, she admitted to be an avid coffee drinker who used to drink more than 5 cups of coffee/day since she was in high-school. She also heard from her colleague that a high level of caffeine contained in coffee could affect women fertility. They did not prefer to undergo medically assisted reproduction and would like to know whether the previously mentioned factor plays an important role in female infertility. The wife asked the doctor whether her high caffeine intake contributes to her infertility status?

INTRODUCTION

Primary infertility can be described by many specific definitions. It is defined as the inability to conceive after 12 months of routine unprotected sexual intercourse without a previous history of conceiving, while also defined as the inability to become pregnant or to carry out the pregnancy to a live birth [1, 2]. It is estimated that infertility has a prevalence of 9 to 18% worldwide, with an estimation of 48.5 million infertile couples in 2010 [1, 3]. Infertility is caused by both male and female factors. Female factors include ovarian disorders (*i.e.* Polycystic ovarian disease (PCOS)), endometriosis, hormonal imbalances, as well as suggested lifestyle factors such as smoking habit, alcohol, and caffeine consumption, and other dietary habits [4].

Female primary infertility can be assessed using laboratory investigations (*i.e.* biopsy and hormonal levels), imaging (*i.e.* hysterosalpingogram), as well as recorded data such as time to pregnancy [3, 5]. Time to pregnancy represents the final outcome of conception expressed in time (*i.e.* 6 or 12 months) rather than quantitative measures of biological processes observed in laboratory investigations such as hormone levels. Time to pregnancy has been proven as a cost-effective, and reliable variable to study infertility [5]. Furthermore, spontaneous abortion has also been used to evaluate primary infertility by various studies as an endpoint in which the female cannot carry out pregnancy [2].

Dietary factor has been suggested to cause infertility, with caffeine intake being one of the subjects. Caffeine (1,3,7-trimethylxanthine) is widely consumed and found mainly in coffee (60-75%), but also in other beverages such as tea, soft drinks, and energy drinks. Moderate caffeine intake has been proposed to have beneficial health effects while excessive caffeine intake (>300-600 mg/day or 4-7 cups/day) may represent health risks, with the reproductive system being one of them [6].

Various studies have shown conflicting results of caffeine impact on various reproductive variables. A study suggests that high caffeine intake affects the free estradiol (E2) hormone, which is important for ovulation. However, the results were conflicting and inconclusive as non-significantly lower and higher free E2 levels were shown depending on race. It is suggested that caffeine affects estrogen metabolism through aromatase inhibition [7]. Furthermore, an animal study suggested that caffeine disrupts oocyte maturation by inhibiting cAMP phosphodiesterase, thus increasing the intracellular cAMP level [8]. These variables, in turn, could cause the inability to conceive, expressed by time to pregnancy. Furthermore, caffeine molecules are small enough to cross the placental barrier, and are suggested to affect endogenous hormone levels such as estradiol and progesterone in the luteal phase, while also increasing sex hormone binding globulin (SHBG) the end product of which can disrupt pregnancy and increase the possibility of spontaneous abortion [9]. Therefore, our aim is to investigate whether daily high caffeine consumption might be associated with primary infertility indicated by time to pregnancy and spontaneous abortion.

METHODS

Literature searching was done based on PubMed and Scopus, using terminologies and filters indexed in Table **1**. Duplicate studies were identified and subsequently removed; the results attained were then screened by titles and abstracts by applying both our inclusion and exclusion criteria and were subsequently checked for their full-text availability. Inclusion criteria were human studies on a female of reproductive age, with selected study designs (systematic review/meta-analysis, cohort, and case-control studies), while exclusion criteria were studies with medically assisted reproduction. Complete readings of those articles were then commenced and suitable articles were chosen accordingly. The searching results are shown in Fig. (**1**). Two independent reviewers assessed the quality of studies by employing the CEBM assessment tool for meta-analysis study, and NOS assessment tool for both cohort and case-control studies.

RESULTS

This evidence-based case report aimed to determine the association between daily high caffeine intake with primary infertility expressed with time to pregnancy (TTP) and spontaneous abortion (SAB) as the primary endpoints. From the literature searching (Fig. **1**), 22 full-text articles were included after the title and abstract screening along with inclusion and exclusion criteria. From those 22 articles, 8 articles were excluded due to unsuitable study designs. From the remaining 14 articles, 10 of them were already included in the meta-analysis, which gave us the final results of 4 articles (2 cohort studies, 1 case-control study, and 1 meta-analysis).

Table 1. Search strategy used in PubMed and Scopus.

Location	Terminology	Filter	Hits
PubMed	("Infertility"[MeSH] OR fertility)) AND (caffeine* OR coffe* OR cola OR tea OR "soft drink"))	human studies, female studies, title and abstract	151
Scopus - Elsevier	(caffeine* OR coffe* OR cola OR tea OR "soft drink") AND (infertility OR fertility)	human studies, female studies, title and abstract	195

A meta-analysis of cohort and case-control studies (n=35) done by Lyngso *et al.* [10] was critically appraised using the CEBM assessment tool, as shown in Table **1**. Subsequently, we conclude the meta-analysis is relevant to the topic and in line with our patient. This meta-analysis aimed to investigate the association between coffee or caffeine intake and fertility, measured through time to pregnancy (TTP) and spontaneous abortion (SAB). In total, 47 studies were included in the review, of which only 35 had dose-response information to intervention and thus eligible to be included in the meta-analysis. Whereas, the remaining 12 studies were only included in the review as a narrative description as it provides insufficient data to be included in the meta-analysis [10].

The meta-analysis of 2 studies that provided sufficient data on TTP reported no clear association between caffeine intake and natural fertility as measured by TTP (p=0.98 for TTP >12 months) ; pooled relative risk 0.99 (95% CI: 0.88, 1.11) for 100 mg caffeine/day group and 0.97 (95% CI: 0.71, 1.33) for 600 mg caffeine/day group in comparison to no caffeine intake. However, due to the small number of studies included in the analysis, the result was not conclusive and should be interpreted with care [10].

Whereas based on the meta-analysis of 27 studies that provided sufficient data on SAB, it was shown that increased caffeine consumption significantly increased the risk of SAB (overall association p < 0.0001); pooled relative risk for SAB was 1.08 (95% CI: 1.03, 1.13) for 100 mg caffeine / day, 1.37 (95% CI: 1.19,1.57) for 300 mg caffeine / day and 2.32 (95% CI: 1.162, 3.31) for 600 mg caffeine/day in comparison to no caffeine [10].

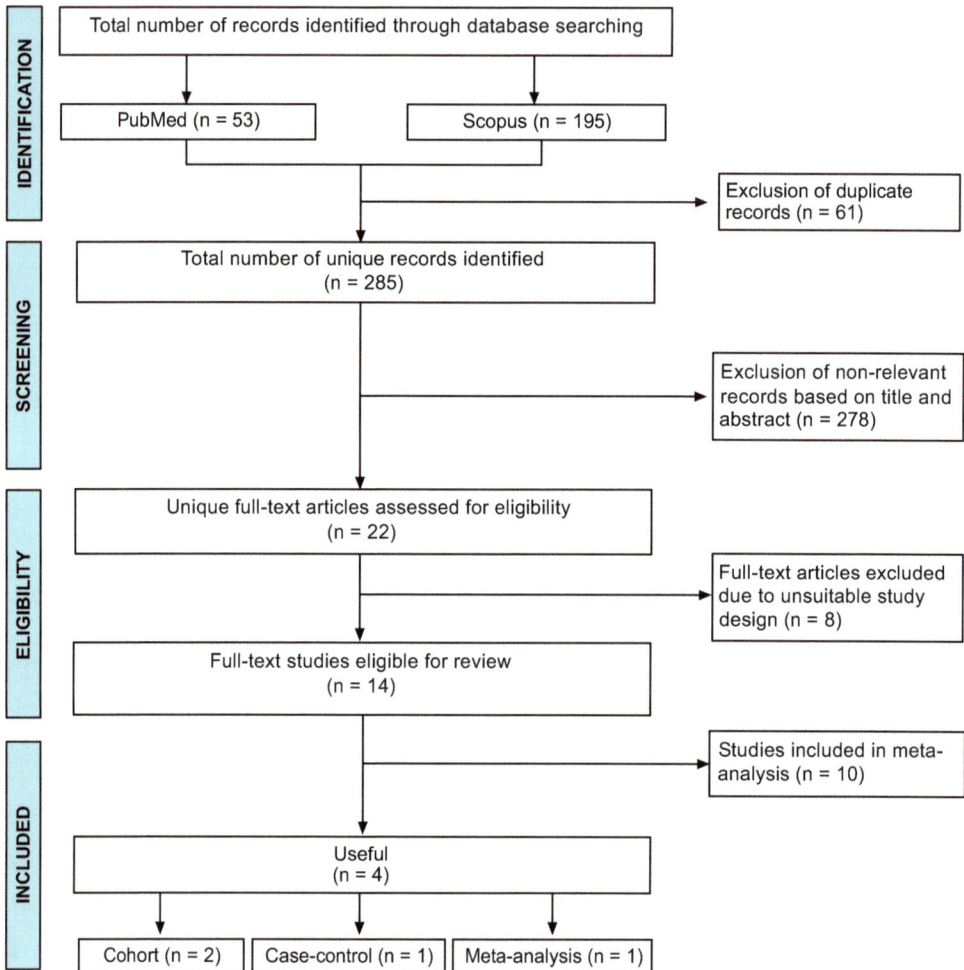

Fig. (1). Search Strategy Flowchart.

Table **2** provides the critical appraisal of two cohort studies published in 2016 and 2018 respectively. Both of the studies were critically appraised; the NOS score revealed a low risk of bias. The study by Wesselink *et al.*, found no significant association between fertility and caffeine intake (RR = 1.10) shown in Table **3** [11]. Having said this, as the source of caffeine varies in this study, they also assess the relationship between individual beverages (*i.e.* coffee, tea, soda) and fecundability. From this individual analysis, it was found that caffeinated black tea was related to a slight reduction in fecundability (RR = 0.89, 95% CI = 0.53-1.48). Regarding this matter, they conclude that compounds other than caffeine contained in each beverage may influence the results of the study [11, 12].

The second study by Soylu *et al.*, also revealed no correlation between caffeine intake and increased risk of primary infertility (RR = 0.99; NNH = 1000) [12]. Individual beverages represented by coffee (HR = 1.00; 95% CI = 0.97–1.03), tea (HR = 1.01; 95% CI = 0.99-1.03) were also not associated with increased risk of primary infertility. The summary of the main finding of each study is provided in Table **3** [12].

Table 2. Critical appraisal results for cohort studies.

Author	Study Population	Level of Evidence	Source of Caffeine	Risk of Bias										Total NOS Score
				Selection (a)				Compara-bility (b)		Exposure/ Outcome (c)				
				1	2	3	4	1	2	1	2	3		
Wesselink *et al.* [11]	2,135 pregnancy planners in North America	2b	Coffee, tea, soda, and energy drinks	*	*		*	*			*	*		6
Soylu *et al.* [12]	7,574 nulliparous Danish women aged 20–29 years	2b	Coffee and tea	*	*		*	*	*	*	*	*		8

(a) Selection: 1. representativeness of the exposed cohort; 2. selection of non-exposed cohort; 3. ascertainment of exposure; 4. demonstration of outcome of interest was not present at the start of the study.
(b) Comparability: 1. comparability of cohort on the basis of the design or analysis; 2. confounding factors controlled.
(c) Exposure/outcome: 1. assessment of outcome; 2. duration of follow up, 3. adequacy of follow up of cohorts.

Besides the systematic review-meta analysis and cohort study described above, we also found one case-control study that has not been included in the systematic review that we used [13]. The study was also critically appraised for the risk of bias (Table **4**), and the main finding is described in Table **5**. This study found that when compared to no caffeine intake, consumption of >300 mg caffeine was related to an increased risk of delayed pregnancy (OR = 1.91) [13]. In addition, this study also demonstrated that the relationship between high caffeine intake and delayed pregnancy is different when adjusted by the smoking status of the women. Despite the satisfying result, it must be noted that the study was prone to recall bias as the subjects were asked to remember their caffeine consumption over a 10 years period before the interview. Based on Newcastle-Ottawa scoring, this case-control study is scored 4, which implied that it is not sufficiently suitable to be used as evidence.

Table 3. Main Findings of cohort studies.

Author	Main Findings	Risk Parameters	
Wesselink *et al.* [11]	There was no significant association between total caffeine intake and fecundability. However, when the effect of each beverage was analyzed individually, only caffeinated black tea intake was found to cause a reduction in fecundability (FR for ≥ 2 *vs.* 0 cups/day black tea=0.89, 95% CI=0.53-1.48).	Exposure Late pregnancy Total (+) (-) High caffeine intake (+) 45 63 108 (-) 772 1255 2027 Total 817 1318 2135	
		CER	772/2027 = 0.38
		EER	45/108 = 0.42
		RR	0.42/0.38 = 1.10
		RD	| 0.38-0.42 | = 0.04
		NNH	1/0.04 = 25
Soylu *et al.* [12]	There was no association between coffee (hazard ratio 1.00; 95% confidence interval (CI), 0.97–1.03), tea (hazard ratio 1.01; 95% CI, 0.99– 1.03) or total caffeine (hazard ratio 1.00; 95% CI 0.98–1.02) consumption and the risk of primary infertility in women.	Exposure Late pregnancy Total (+) (-) High caffeine intake (+) 465 3792 4257 (-) 357 2960 3317 Total 822 6752 7574	
		CER	357/3317 = 0.108
		EER	465/4257 = 0.109
		RR	0.108/0.1091 = 0.99
		RD	| 0.108-0.109 | = 0.001
		NNH	1/0.001 = 1000

CER= control event rate; EER = experimental event rate; RR = relative risk; RD = risk difference; NNH = number needed to harm

Table 4. Critical appraisal results of case-control study.

Author	Study Population	Level of Evidence	Source of Caffeine	Selection (a)				Comparability (b)		Exposure/ Outcome (c)			Total NOS Score
				1	2	3	4	1	2	1	2	3	
Stanton CK *et al.*, 1995 [13]	Effects of caffeine consumption on delayed conception	3b	Coffee, tea, and soft drink	*		*		*			*		4

(a) Selection: 1. Adequacy of case definition; 2. representativeness of the cases; 3. selection of controls; 3. definition of controls.
(b) Comparability: 1. comparability of cases and controls on the basis of the design or analysis; 3. confounding factors controlled.
(c) Exposure: 1. ascertainment of exposure; 2. same method of ascertainment for cases and controls; 3. non-response rate.

Table 5. The main findings of case-control study.

Author	Main Finding	Risk Parameters			
Stanton CK *et al.*, 1995 [13]	This study found that consumption of more than 300 mg caffeine intake per day increased the risk of delayed conception (Odds Ratio = 1.83, 95% CI 1.13-2.97) compared to women with no caffeine intake at all. However, they also found that this effect of caffeine varied by the smoking status of the women.				

Within Risk Parameters:

Exposure		Late Pregnancy		Total
		(+)	(-)	
High caffeine intake (>300 mg)	(+)	28	145	173
	(-)	208	2110	2318
Total		236	2255	2491

OR*	28 x 2110 / 208 x 145 = 1.96
PEER	208/2318 = 0.09
NNH	[(0.09 x (1.96-1) + 1] / (0.09 x (1.96-1) x (1 – PEER)) = 13.9

OR = odds ratio; PEER = patient expected event rate; NNH = number needed to harm

DISCUSSION

Caffeine consumption has been thought to be correlated with numerous health issues in pregnant women. The World Health Organization (WHO) mentioned that pregnant women should avoid caffeine consumption of more than 300 mg per day [14]. From our search strategy, we found one meta-analysis, two cohorts, as well as one case-control study that aimed to describe the relationship between primary infertility and excessive consumption.

Although results of meta-analysis of cohort studies revealed that excessive consumption is related to increased risk of SAB, significant heterogeneity was detected ($I^2 = 73.7\%$, p<0.0001) and Egger's regression test revealed a substantial publication bias (p<0.0001). When stratified and reanalyzed on caffeine consumption, adjustment status, study quality, and study design, significant heterogeneity was only found between different study designs in which association was more pronounced in cohort studies in comparison to case-control studies. Furthermore, studies not reporting any association between caffeine intake and SAB might not be included resulting in a publication bias. In the studies included in the meta-analysis, the definition of high caffeine intake and low caffeine intake between treatment and control group differs, thus the use of the dose-response analysis is appropriate as it allows a more detailed and flexible description of caffeine consumption and its effect on primary fertility over a range of exposure [10].

It has been postulated that due to the small size of caffeine molecules, it passes freely through the placenta, making both mother and the fetus exposed to the same caffeine levels. Coffee intake has also been affiliated with decreased estrogen and hCG levels in pregnant mothers [15]. Caffeine can also increase blood catecholamine levels which may interfere with placental blood flow. These suggested mechanisms may help to explain the relationship between increased risk of SAB and high levels of caffeine intake, as observed in the meta-analysis [16].

On the other hand, both cohort studies indicated no association between total caffeine intake and reduced female fecundability measured as time to pregnancy [11, 12]. However, Wesselink *et al.*, suggested that only caffeinated tea caused a slight reduction in female fecundability [11]. But, this association is weak (RR = 0.85, 95% CI = 0.58-1.25) and questionable as they also found a slight reduction in fecundability in those females who drink decaffeinated tea (RR = 0.82, 95% CI = 0,65-1,03), suggesting that other compounds in tea may play a role in reducing female fecundability [11]. Another possibility is that other confounding factors may have influenced fecundability, such as genetic factors and prior health issues that were not adjusted in the study. On a positive note, the prospective evaluation of the patient's dietary intake in this study reduces the possibility of information bias.

Soylu *et al.*, in their study used a large sample (n = 7574) and assessed fertility based on a nationwide registry instead of self-report, which increased the validity of the study [12]. However, we have identified several weaknesses of this study. Firstly, they did not adjust for body mass index due to data unavailability for approximately 70% of the subjects. BMI could be an important confounding factor for female infertility, as shown in previous studies, as excessive fat could produce more estrogen and interfere in the ovulation cycle, as well as related to pregnancy complications such as gestational diabetes, pre-eclampsia, and stillbirth [17, 18]. Secondly, the study excluded a large number of women with missing information (n=1567), thus it may cause selection bias [12]. Thirdly, they only accounted for coffee and tea, whereas other caffeinated beverages such as soft drink may also be linked to female infertility.

Different from the cohort study, a case-control study reports that high caffeine consumption is significantly related to a higher risk of delayed pregnancy, which is the indicator of primary infertility [13]. Having said this, it is important to note that this study uses a case-control design, which is not the most preferred design of study for etiology research. Also, this study is prone to recall bias as subjects were asked to mention their caffeine intake for over a 10 years period. To add, considering caffeine consumption during the first month of pregnancy to reflect the pre-pregnancy consumption may lead to misclassification of caffeine consumption as pregnant women might change their caffeine intake during this time.

Caffeine may affect fecundity endpoints through several proposed hypotheses, albeit the exact mechanism still needs further elucidations. Inside the body, caffeine acts as a non-selective adenosine agonist, which increases the c-AMP concentration resulting in altered levels of blood catecholamines. Aside from being both neuroendocrine and cardiovascular stimulant, which may indirectly influence the reproductive system, some studies also demonstrated the detrimental effects of caffeine on estradiol levels [19]. This is in accordance with other studies that reported the association between caffeine and increased sex hormone-binding globulin levels. The altered reproductive hormone levels may interfere with ovulation and corpus luteum functioning, contributing to subfecundity [20].

However, other studies showed contradicting results, which reported that high levels of caffeine consumption caused increased or no effects on estradiol levels. Another plausible pathway involved is the CYP1A2 hepatic enzyme, which metabolizes both estradiol and caffeine, thus caffeine may interfere with estradiol levels through a common metabolism pathway [21]. Of note, other substances contained in coffee, such as lignans and isoflavonoids, belonging to the phytoestrogen family, may strongly bind with the estrogen receptor. Consequently, the menstrual cycle could be affected due to increased estradiol levels, as one study reports that >300 mg/day consumption of caffeine is linked to a shorter menstrual cycle period [13]. These contradictory results support the suggestion that caffeine intake, regardless of the amount, does not have any putative effect with fecundity outcomes.

CONCLUSION

Overall, studies show a non-significant association between high caffeine consumption and time to pregnancy as a parameter of primary infertility, on the contrary, the meta-analysis show that high caffeine consumption is related to SAB. However, heterogeneity of results in the meta-analysis must be considered in which results must be used with caution. Hence, we conclude that high caffeine is not associated with female primary infertility and that restriction of the consumption of caffeine is not necessarily needed in women trying to achieve pregnancy.

CONSENT FOR PUBLICATION

Not Applicable.

CONFLICT OF INTEREST

The author declares no conflict of interest, financial or otherwise.

ACKNOWLEDGEMENTS

Declared none.

REFERENCES

[1]   Anwar SAA. Infertility: A review on causes, treatment and management. Women's Health Gynecol 2016; 2: 6.

[2]   Mascarenhas MN, Flaxman SR, Boerma T, Vanderpoel S, Stevens GA. National, regional, and global trends in infertility prevalence since 1990: a systematic analysis of 277 health surveys. PLoS Med 2012; 9(12): e1001356.
[http://dx.doi.org/10.1371/journal.pmed.1001356] [PMID: 23271957]

[3]   Hanson B, Johnstone E, Dorais J, Silver B, Peterson CM, Hotaling J. Female infertility, infertility-associated diagnoses, and comorbidities: a review. J Assist Reprod Genet 2017; 34(2): 167-77.
[http://dx.doi.org/10.1007/s10815-016-0836-8] [PMID: 27817040]

[4]   Healy DL, Trounson AO, Andersen AN. Female infertility: causes and treatment. Lancet 1994; 343(8912): 1539-44.
[http://dx.doi.org/10.1016/S0140-6736(94)92941-6] [PMID: 7911874]

[5]   Joffe M. Time to pregnancy: a measure of reproductive function in either sex. Asclepios Project. Occup Environ Med 1997; 54(5): 289-95.
[http://dx.doi.org/10.1136/oem.54.5.289] [PMID: 9196448]

[6]   Nawrot P, Jordan S, Eastwood J, Rotstein J, Hugenholtz A, Feeley M. Effects of caffeine on human health. Food Addit Contam 2003; 20(1): 1-30.
[http://dx.doi.org/10.1080/0265203021000007840] [PMID: 12519715]

[7]   Schliep KC, Schisterman EF, Mumford SL, *et al.* Caffeinated beverage intake and reproductive hormones among premenopausal women in the BioCycle Study. Am J Clin Nutr 2012; 95(2): 488-97.
[http://dx.doi.org/10.3945/ajcn.111.021287] [PMID: 22237060]

[8]   Miao YL, Shi LH, Lei ZL, *et al.* Effects of caffeine on *in vivo* and *in vitro* oocyte maturation in mice. Theriogenology 2007; 68(4): 640-5.
[http://dx.doi.org/10.1016/j.theriogenology.2007.04.061] [PMID: 17576000]

[9]   Hahn KA, Wise LA, Rothman KJ, *et al.* Caffeine and caffeinated beverage consumption and risk of spontaneous abortion. Hum Reprod 2015; 30(5): 1246-55.
[http://dx.doi.org/10.1093/humrep/dev063] [PMID: 25788567]

[10]   Lyngsø J, Ramlau-Hansen CH, Bay B, Ingerslev HJ, Hulman A, Kesmodel US. Association between coffee or caffeine consumption and fecundity and fertility: a systematic review and dose-response meta-analysis. Clin Epidemiol 2017; 9: 699-719.
[http://dx.doi.org/10.2147/CLEP.S146496] [PMID: 29276412]

[11]   Wesselink AK, Wise LA, Rothman KJ, *et al.* Caffeine and caffeinated beverage consumption and fecundability in a preconception cohort. Reprod Toxicol 2016; 62: 39-45.
[http://dx.doi.org/10.1016/j.reprotox.2016.04.022] [PMID: 27112524]

[12] Í Soylu L, Jensen A, Juul KE, *et al.* Coffee, tea and caffeine consumption and risk of primary infertility in women: a Danish cohort study. Acta Obstet Gynecol Scand 2018; 97(5): 570-6.
[http://dx.doi.org/10.1111/aogs.13307] [PMID: 29364517]

[13] Stanton CK, Gray RH. Effects of caffeine consumption on delayed conception. Am J Epidemiol 1995; 142(12): 1322-9.
[http://dx.doi.org/10.1093/oxfordjournals.aje.a117600] [PMID: 7503053]

[14] WHO recommendation on caffeine intake during pregnancy. The WHO Reproductive Health Library. Geneva: World Health Organization 2016.

[15] Aldridge A, Bailey J, Neims AH. The disposition of caffeine during and after pregnancy. Semin Perinatol 1981; 5(4): 310-4.
[PMID: 7302604]

[16] Lawson CC, LeMasters GK, Levin LS, Liu JH. Pregnancy hormone metabolite patterns, pregnancy symptoms, and coffee consumption. Am J Epidemiol 2002; 156(5): 428-37.
[http://dx.doi.org/10.1093/aje/kwf035] [PMID: 12196312]

[17] Siega-Riz A-M, Siega-Riz A-M, Laraia B. The implications of maternal overweight and obesity on the course of pregnancy and birth outcomes. Matern Child Health J 2006; 10(5) (Suppl.): S153-6.
[http://dx.doi.org/10.1007/s10995-006-0115-x] [PMID: 16927160]

[18] Robinson HE, O'Connell CM, Joseph KS, McLeod NL. Maternal outcomes in pregnancies complicated by obesity. Obstet Gynecol 2005; 106(6): 1357-64.
[http://dx.doi.org/10.1097/01.AOG.0000188387.88032.41] [PMID: 16319263]

[19] Bellet S, Roman L, DeCastro O, Kim KE, Kershbaum A. Effect of coffee ingestion on catecholamine release. Metabolism 1969; 18(4): 288-91.
[http://dx.doi.org/10.1016/0026-0495(69)90049-3] [PMID: 5777013]

[20] Lane JD, Steege JF, Rupp SL, Kuhn CM. Menstrual cycle effects on caffeine elimination in the human female. Eur J Clin Pharmacol 1992; 43(5): 543-6.
[http://dx.doi.org/10.1007/BF02285099] [PMID: 1483492]

[21] Sata F, Yamada H, Suzuki K, *et al.* Caffeine intake, CYP1A2 polymorphism and the risk of recurrent pregnancy loss. Mol Hum Reprod 2005; 11(5): 357-60.
[http://dx.doi.org/10.1093/molehr/gah175] [PMID: 15849225]

CHAPTER 4

An Overview of *Urena sinuata*: Phytochemistry and Pharmacological Activities

Pranta Ray[1], Rajib Hossain[1], Md. Matiur Rahman[2] and Muhammad Torequl Islam[1,*]

[1] *Department of Pharmacy, Life Science Faculty, Bangabandhu Sheikh Mujibur Rahman Science and Technology University, Gopalganj (Dhaka)-8100, Bangladesh*

[2] *Department of Pharmacy, Ranada Prasad Shaha University, Narayanganj-1400, Bangladesh*

Abstract: Urena genus consists of two species named *Urena lobata* L. and *Urena sinuata* L. These plants have various pharmacological properties, including antioxidant, anti-diarrheal, anti-parasitic, anti-inflammatory and analgesic activities and a variety of phytochemicals. *U. sinuata* is a medicinal herb, which is frequently used by the traditional practitioners in Bangladesh, India and many other countries of the world for the treatment of various diseases. The plant roots are anti-rheumatic, anti-pyretic, emollient, refrigerant, maturant, and act as a cooling agent. In this study, we summarize a detailed overview of the *U. sinuata* based on the most recent available literature (till Jun 2020). Findings suggest that *U. sinuata* possesses many important phytochemical and pharmacological activities. According to scientific reports, *U. sinuata* possesses carbohydrates and gums, reducing sugars, alkaloids, steroids, glycosides and flavonoids. Pharmacological investigations suggest that the plant has antioxidant, anti-diarrheal, anti-inflammatory, anti-pyretic, anxiolytic, analgesic, sedative, thrombolytic, insecticidal and repellent activities. In conclusion, *U. sinuata* may be one of the best sources of plant-based drugs.

Keywords: Pharmacological activities, Phytochemicals, *Urena sinuata*.

INTRODUCTION

Urena sinuata L. (Family: Malvaceae) (Fig. **1**) is also known as a sub-species of *U. lobata* [1, 2]. In Venezuelan folk medicine, Urena plant species have been utilized for their pharmacological properties, which include- anti-bacterial [3], anti-diarrheal [4], anti-parasitic [5], anti-inflammatory and analgesic [6] activities. It has been reported that a variety of compounds are isolated from this species,

* **Corresponding author Muhammad Torequl Islam:** Department of Pharmacy, Life Science Faculty, Bangabandhu Sheikh Mujibur Rahman Science and Technology University, Gopalganj (Dhaka)-8100, Bangladesh; Tel: +88026682257; Fax: +88026682173; E-mail: dmt.islam@bsmrstu.edu.bd

Anna Capasso (Ed.)

including steroids (*i.e.*, *β*-sitosterol) [7], xanthones [8], flavonoids (*e.g.*, luteolin, hypolaetin, quercetin, gossypetin, kaempferol, apigenin and chrysoeriol) and fatty acids [2].

U. sinuata is a medicinal herb locally known as 'Kunjia' in Bangladesh and has a good reputation in Bangladesh, India and many other countries of the world [9]. *U. sinuata*, also known as *U. lobata* or *U. morifolia*, is a wild shrubby plant widely grown throughout the world in tropical and subtropical areas with many important folk medicinal usages [10, 11].

The plant roots are anti-rheumatic, anti-pyretic, sweet, and slightly cooling [12]. In Brazil, its stems are used in severe windy colic [13] alongside the root decoction that is used in dysentery, rheumatic pains, and tonsillitis [11] and the roots, in India, are used as an external application for lumbago and in the Pacific, Trinidad and Tobago, China and India, for reproductive purposes for both genders [14]. The roots are also considered as emollient, refrigerant and maturant in the Philippines [15, 16] and in dry and inveterate chronic coughs, the plant flowers are used as an expectorant [11]. The infusion of the flowers is used for gargles and throat bronchitis [17]. The leaves of the plant are prescribed in inflammation of the intestines and bladder. The whole plant is considered not only medicinal, but also an economic plant for various purposes in Madagascar, Nigeria and Western Sudan, Chad, Central African Republic, Zaire and Gabon for producing fiber (Aramina fiber) [15, 16].

This paper offers an up to date summary of the phytochemical and pharmacological properties of the *U. sinuata* on the basis of the database (*e.g.*, PubMed, Science Direct and Google Scholar) reports till Jun 2020.

RESEARCH METHODOLOGY

The literature on *U. sinuata* botanical description, secondary metabolites, biological properties were collected, analyzed and summarized in this review. Scientific search engines such as PubMed, ScienceDirect, SpringerLink, Web of Science, Scopus, Wiley Online, Scifnder, and Google Scholar, and various patient offices (*e.g.*, WIPO, CIPO, USPTO) were used to collect all published articles about this species. The common keyword '*Urena sinuata*', alone or paired with the 'chemical compounds', and 'pharmacological activities'. No language restrictions were imposed. The identification and manipulation of the collected data were based on their titles, abstracts and contents. Reference lists of the retrieved papers were also examined to identify further relevant papers. Chemical structures were drawn by using the Chemsketch version 12.01 software.

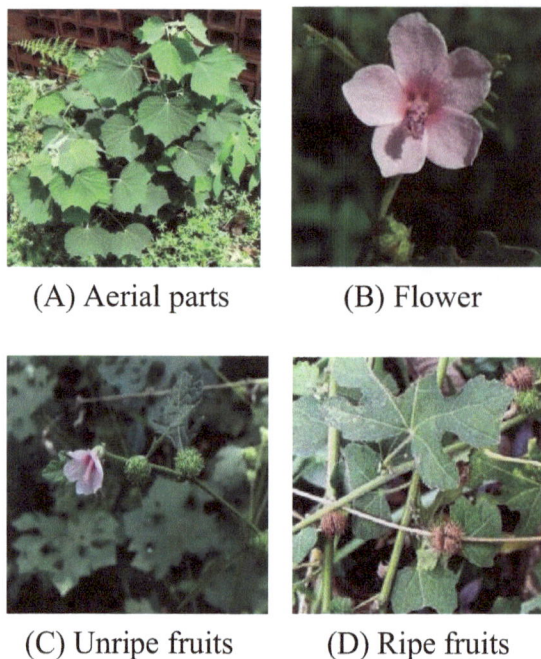

(A) Aerial parts   (B) Flower

(C) Unripe fruits   (D) Ripe fruits

Fig. (1). Images of different parts of *Urena sinuata* L.

FINDINGS

Phytochemicals of *U. Sinuata*

The plant contains carbohydrates and gums, reducing sugars, alkaloids, steroids, glycosides and flavonoids [9, 18]. Sosa and Rosquete [6] isolated and identified three quercetagetin glucosides from the leaves of the *U. sinuata*. In this study, quercetagetin-6, 7-*O*-dimethylether-3-β-D-glucopyranoside (**I**), quercetagetin-6, 7-*O*-dimethylether-4'-β-D glucopyranoside (**II**), and quercetagetin-6, 7-*O* dimethylether-3'-β-D-gluco-pyranoside (**III**) (Fig. **2**) were the major flavonoids. In another study, Sosa *et al.* [2], also report that the plant contains 6,7-di-*O*-methyl-quercetagetin- 3-*O*-β-D-glucopyranoside dihydrate (**I**).

Pharmacological Activities of *U. Sinuata*

Antioxidant Activity

In the cell, an antioxidant can temper the negative influence of free radicals and associated reactions [19]. Block [20] reports that antioxidants have potential activity in reducing cancer risk. Saha and Paul [9] reported that chloroform extract of the *U. sinuata* showed an antioxidant capacity (2, 2-diphenyl-1-picrylhydrazyl (DPPH) assay at 20-800 µg/ml; IC_{50}: 10.64 µg/ml).

Anti-Diarrhoeal Activity

In developing countries, diarrheal disease is often a leading source of morbidity and mortality, especially among children causing a major healthcare problem [21]. Microorganisms serve as major causative agents of diarrhea in humans that include *Shigella flexneri*, *Staphylococcus aureus*, *Escherichia coli*, *Salmonella typhi*, *Aeromonas hydrophila*, and *Plesiomonas shigelloides* [22 - 24]. Urena plant species have anti-diarrheal activity [4]. In humans, *Candida albicans* has also been recognized to cause diarrhea characterized by a discharge of semi-solid or watery fecal matter in the bowels three or even more times every day [25, 26]. In a study, different fractions of *U. sinuata* leaf (200 and 400 mg/kg, p.o.) were found to exert a potential anti-diarrhoeal effect on Albino Wistar rats (*Rattus norvigicus*) [27].

Anti-Nociceptive Activity

Emran *et al.* [18], demonstrated that the chloroform extract of the *U. sinuata* leaves exhibited anti-nociceptive activity in the formalin-induced writhing mouse model. The test showed that at 400 mg/kg (p.o.), chloroform extract of the *U. sinuata* significantly attenuated writhing reflex (37.39% and 65.98% at 1st phase, and last phase, respectively). At the same time, diclofenac inhibited 47.27% (at 10 mg/kg) in the last phase.

In the glutamate-induced test, it has been observed that the chloroform extract of the *U. sinuata* leaves significantly ameliorated the noxious stimuli. At the dose of 400 mg/kg, it induced 88.68% inhibition of the nociception that was higher than the reference drug (diclofenac sodium creates 58.32% inhibition of the pain) [18].

Anti-Inflammatory Activity

In paw, carrageenan produced inflammatory edema, which increased gradually. The chloroform extract of *U. sinuata* leaves exerted a significant anti-inflammatory effect at 200 and 400 mg/kg (i.p.) doses in carrageenan-induced rat paw edema. The reference drug (diclofenac sodium) showed an anti-inflammatory effect of at 10 mg/kg (i.p.). The effects of the extract on the proliferative phase of inflammation were significantly attenuated at 200 and 400 mg/kg (b.w.) dose in cotton pellet-induced granuloma rats [18].

Anti-Pyretic Activity

The chloroform extract of *U. sinuata* leaves reduced the body temperature of the experimental animals. In a study, at 400 mg/kg (b.w.), the chloroform leaf extract of *U. sinuata* significantly ameliorated the body temperature (up to 4 h) from 37.57 to 36.29 °C [18].

Insecticidal and Insect-Repellent Activities

Abdullah *et al.* [12], conducted the insecticidal and insect repellent tests with the chloroform extracts of fruit, leaf, root and stem of the plant against the adult *Tribolium castaneum* (red flour beetle), suggesting that the leaf, root and stem extracts exerted better toxic effects than the fruit extract.

Thrombolytic Activity

Thrombosis is the blockage of blood vessels with clots, which can lead to acute myocardial infarction and ischemic stroke and it has been reported as one of the leading causes of death [28]. For thrombosis, the administration of thrombolytic agents to dissolve the blood clot is the only treatment available [29]. All over the world for the treatment of this disease, the thrombolytic agents that comprise tissue plasminogen activator (t-PA), urokinase (UK), streptokinase (SK), *etc.* are extensively used [28].

Mannan *et al.* [30], investigated the thrombolytic activity of plant extracts, by applying an *in vitro* thrombolytic method, in blood sample from healthy human volunteers, suggesting the aqueous extract of the *U. sinuata* showed a mild thrombolytic effect in comparison to the standard drug streptokinase. The thrombolytic activity of the chloroform extract of *U. sinuata* was also reported by Saha and Swati [31]. Moreover, Emran *et al.* [28], also reported thrombolytic effects of the herb.

Sedative, Anxiolytic, and Analgesic Activities

The crude methanolic leaf extract of the *U. sinuata* (400 mg/kg, p.o.) is evident to exert a significant sedative effect in mice [11]. Another study showed that the chloroform extract of the *U. sinuata* leaves exerted neuropharmacological effects in rodents. The chloroform extract of *U. Sinuata*, at doses 200 and 400 mg/kg (p.o.) reduced the locomotion activity in hole cross and open field test [18]. In the thiopental sodium induced sleeping test, the extract at 200 and 400 mg/kg doses exhibited a significant attenuation of the time of inception of sleep. The effect of chloroform leaf extract of *U. sinuata* (200 and 400 mg/kg) was similar to that of the standard drug (thiopental sodium). Both doses of the extract increased the duration of sleeping time in experimental animals [18].

The plant extract was also found to exert an analgesic effect on the experimental animals. The chloroform leaf extract of *U. sinuata* showed an analgesic effect at 200 and 400 mg/kg (p.o.) in hot plate, acetic acid-induced writhing, and tail immersion models in rodents [18].

TOXICOLOGICAL PROFILE

The chloroform extract of *U. sinuata* leaves did not cause mortality, behavioral changes like sedation, excitability, *etc.* or allergic manifestations after oral administration at various doses and during the 8 h observation period after administration [18].

DISCUSSION

Several studies on this medicinal plant suggest that this plant has antioxidant, anti-diarrheal, anti-inflammatory, anti-nociceptive, anti-pyretic, anxiolytic, analgesic, insecticidal and insect repellent, and sedative effects.

The phytochemical screening of the crude extract and the active fraction of *U. sinuata* contains carbohydrates, alkaloids, flavonoids, glycosides, tannins, and saponins. *U. sinuata* exhibited many important biological activities in several test systems that may be due to the presence of chemical constituents, flavonoids, alkaloids, glycosides, tannins, and saponins. Unfortunately, to date, only three flavonoids (Fig. **2**) were isolated by Sosa and Rosquete [6] and Sosa *et al.* [2], from this plant. It has been seen that phytochemicals, including tannins, flavonoids, alkaloids, sterols, terpenes, and resins, have significant anti-nociceptive, sedative, and anti-psychotic effects [32].

The plant extracts were also seen to exert greater activities on the test systems than the standard drugs. For example, the crude extract showed anti-inflammatory effect better than diclofenac sodium; anxiolytic and sedative effects better than thiopental sodium. Moreover, the plant also reduced the locomotion activity in experimental animals.

The DPPH assay is potent for identifying the antioxidant activity of diverse components, including plant extracts [33]. *U. sinuata* also showed a concentration-dependent antioxidant effect in this assay. Furthermore, it exhibited anti-diarrheal, analgesic, insecticidal and insect repellent activities in several systems. In view of these findings, more research is necessary to explore and characterize the chemical compounds and their pharmacological and toxicological aspects of this hopeful medicinal herb.

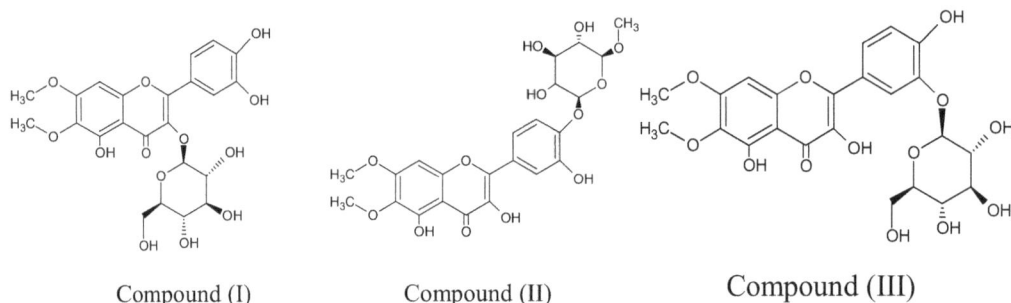

Compound (I)	Compound (II)	Compound (III)

Fig. (2). Chemical structures of isolated and identified three quercetagetin glucosides from *Urena sinuata* L.

SUMMARY AND PERSPECTIVES

Findings suggest that *U. sinuata* possesses a number of bioactive compounds and has various important pharmacological activities. Its antioxidant, anti-inflammatory, sedative and analgesic activities suggest that the herb has a neuroprotective effect. Generally, the antioxidants are protective in nature. Antioxidant, anti-inflammatory and anti-atherothrombosis activities may be linked to its cardioprotective effects. Alkaloids, glycosides, and flavonoids are known for their diverse biological activities. In addition, the leaf extract of *U. sinuata* and its fractions showed an anti-diarrheal effect, while the chloroform extracts of fruit, leaf, root and stem showed an insecticidal effect against *T. castaneum*. However, the scientific reports on this exceptional medicinal herb are not sufficient. Therefore, we must conclude by saying that more research works are necessary for this medicinal plant.

CONSENT FOR PUBLICATION

Not Applicable.

CONFLICT OF INTEREST

The author declares no conflict of interest, financial or otherwise.

ACKNOWLEDGEMENTS

Declared none.

REFERENCES

[1]   Valderas JM. Relectura de las Disertaciones de Cavanilles. Collectanea Botanica 1991; 20: 183-238.
        [http://dx.doi.org/10.3989/collectbot.1991.v20.108]

[2]   Sosa A, Rosquete C, Bruno J, *et al.* Crystal Structure Analysis of 6, 7-di-O-Methyl-Quercetage-
        in-3-OBD-Glucopyranoside dihydrate Isolated from *Urena sinuata* L. Avances en Química 2011; 6:
        55-9.

[3]   Mazumder UK, Gupta M, Manikandan L, Bhattacharya S. Antibacterial activity of *Urena lobata* root.
        Fitoterapia 2001; 72(8): 927-9.
        [http://dx.doi.org/10.1016/S0367-326X(01)00330-6] [PMID: 11731119]

[4]   Yadav AK, Tangpu V. Antidiarrheal Activity of *Lithocarpus dealbata* and *Urena lobata*. Extracts:
        Therapeutic Implications. Pharm Biol 2007; 45: 223-9.
        [http://dx.doi.org/10.1080/13880200701213153]

[5]   Nguyen-Pouplin J, Tran H, Tran H, *et al.* Antimalarial and cytotoxic activities of
        ethnopharmacologically selected medicinal plants from South Vietnam. J Ethnopharmacol 2007;
        109(3): 417-27.
        [http://dx.doi.org/10.1016/j.jep.2006.08.011] [PMID: 17010546]

[6]   Sosa A, Rosquete C. Flavonoids from *Urena sinuata* L. Avances en Química 2010; 5: 95-8.

[7]   Lin S, Pan T, Horg C. Chemical constituents of *Urena lobata* L. var. tomentosa (Blume) Walp
        (Malvaceae). Hua Hsueh 1983; 41: 72-3.

[8]   Srinivasan KK, Subramanian SS. Isolation of mangiferin from *Urena lobata.* Arogya 1981; 7: 140-1.

[9]   Saha D, Paul S. Phytochemical screening and *in vitro* antioxidant activity of chloroform extract of
        Urena Sinuata L. Int J Pharm Res Innovat 2013; 6: 19-24.

[10]   Ghani A. Medicinal Plants of Bangladesh. 2nd Revised., Dhaka, Bangladesh: the Asiatic Society of
        Bangladesh 2003.

[11]   Emran TB, Rahman MA. Sedative, anxiolytic and analgesic effects of *Urena sinuata* L. leaf extract in
        animal models. Int Food Res J 2014; 21: 2069-75.

[12]   Abdullah M, Pk AK, Saleh DKMA, Khan AR, Islam N. Insecticidal and repellent activities of the
        chloroform extracts of *Urena sinuata* L. against Triboliumcastaneum (Herbst) adults. Univ J Zool
        Rajshahi Univ 2011; 30: 25-8.
        [http://dx.doi.org/10.3329/ujzru.v30i0.10740]

[13]   Browner CH. Plants used for reproductive health in Oaxaca, Mexico. Econ Bot 1985; 39(4): 482-504.
        [http://dx.doi.org/10.1007/BF02858757] [PMID: 12342712]

[14]   Nadkarni KM. The Indian MateriaMedica, with Ayurvedic, Unani and Home Remedies. Revised and
        enlarged by A.K. Nadkarni. Bombay: Bombay popular Prakashan PVP 1954; pp. 947-8.

[15]   Anon . *The Wealth of India."* –a dictionary of Indian raw materials and industrial prodcuts. CSIR,
        New Delhi 1976; 10: 414-6.

[16]   Ahmed ZU, Begum ZT, Hassan MA, *et al.* Encyclopedia of flora and fauna of Bangladesh. Dhaka:
        Asiatic Society of Bangladesh, 2008.

[17]   Kirtikar KR, Basu BD. Indian Medicinal Plants. 2nd. Allahabad, India: Basu, L.M 1965; pp. 3:1606-
        1609.

[18]   Emran T B, Ahmed S, Zahan S, *et al.* Sedative, anxiolytic, antinociceptive, anti-inflammatory and
        antipyretic effects of a chloroform extract from the leaves of *Urena sinuata* in rodents. J Appl Biol Sci
        2018; 1-19.

[19]   Packer L. Oxidants, antioxidant nutrients and the athlete. J Sports Sci 1997; 15(3): 353-63.
        [http://dx.doi.org/10.1080/026404197367362] [PMID: 9232561]

[20]   Block G. The data support a role for antioxidants in reducing cancer risk. Nutr Rev 1992; 50(7): 207-13.
[http://dx.doi.org/10.1111/j.1753-4887.1992.tb01329.x] [PMID: 1641203]

[21]   Chitme HR, Chandra M, Kaushik S. Studies on anti-diarrhoeal activity of Calotropis gigantea R.Br. in experimental animals. J Pharm Pharm Sci 2004; 7(1): 70-5.
[PMID: 15144737]

[22]   Brenden RA, Miller MA, Janda JM. Clinical disease spectrum and pathogenic factors associated with Plesiomonas shigelloides infections in humans. Rev Infect Dis 1988; 10(2): 303-16.
[http://dx.doi.org/10.1093/clinids/10.2.303] [PMID: 3287561]

[23]   Janda JM, Abbott SL. The genus Aeromonas: taxonomy, pathogenicity, and infection. Clin Microbiol Rev 2010; 23(1): 35-73.
[http://dx.doi.org/10.1128/CMR.00039-09] [PMID: 20065325]

[24]   Umer S, Tekewe A, Kebede N. Antidiarrhoeal and antimicrobial activity of *Calpurnia aurea* leaf extract. BMC Complement Altern Med 2013; 13: 21.
[http://dx.doi.org/10.1186/1472-6882-13-21] [PMID: 23351272]

[25]   Hirschhorn N. The treatment of acute diarrhea in children. An historical and physiological perspective. Am J Clin Nutr 1980; 33(3): 637-63.
[http://dx.doi.org/10.1093/ajcn/33.3.637] [PMID: 6766662]

[26]   Snyder JD, Merson MH. The magnitude of the global problem of acute diarrhoeal disease: a review of active surveillance data. Bull World Health Organ 1982; 60(4): 605-13.
[PMID: 6982783]

[27]   Rahman MS, Sultan RA, Emran TB. Evaluation of the anti-diarrheal activity of methanol extract and its fractions of *Urena sinuata* L. (Borss) leaves. J Appl Pharm Sci 6: 56-60.

[28]   Emran TB, Rahman MA, Uddin MMN, *et al.* Effects of organic extracts and their different fractions of five Bangladeshi plants on *in vitro* thrombolysis. BMC Complement Altern Med 2015; 15: 128.
[http://dx.doi.org/10.1186/s12906-015-0643-2] [PMID: 25902818]

[29]   Kunamneni A, Abdelghani TTA, Ellaiah P. Streptokinase--the drug of choice for thrombolytic therapy. J Thromb Thrombolysis 2007; 23(1): 9-23.
[http://dx.doi.org/10.1007/s11239-006-9011-x] [PMID: 17111203]

[30]   Mannan A, Ahmed AA, Sharmin F, Fatema T, Sikder MOF. *In vitro* thrombolytic assay of *Alpinia zerumbet, Alpinia nigra* and *Urena sinuata*. Int J Res Phytochem Pharmacol 2011; 1: 187-91.

[31]   Saha D, Swati P. Phytochemical screening and the thrombolytic activity of chloroform extract of *Urena sinuata* (L.). J Fundam. Appl Sci (Basel) 2014; 6: 208-19.

[32]   Duke JA. Handbook of phytochemical constituent grass, herbs and other economic plants. Boca Raton, Florida: CRC press 1992.

[33]   Xie J, Schaich KM. Re-evaluation of the 2,2-diphenyl-1-picrylhydrazyl free radical (DPPH) assay for antioxidant activity. J Agric Food Chem 2014; 62(19): 4251-60.
[http://dx.doi.org/10.1021/jf500180u] [PMID: 24738928]

CHAPTER 5

Anti-CHIKV Activities of Diterpenes and Their Derivatives

Muhammad Torequl Islam[*]

Department of Pharmacy, Life Science Faculty, Bangabandhu Sheikh Mujibur Rahman Science and Technology University, Gopalganj (Dhaka)-8100, Bangladesh

Abstract:

Background: Chikungunya (CHIKV) is a mosquito-borne viral disease first described during an outbreak in southern Tanzania in 1952. It is an RNA virus, belonging to the alphavirus genus of the family Togaviridae. To date, CHIKV has been identified in over 60 countries in Asia, Africa, Europe and the Americas. Diterpenes consist of two terpene units, often with the molecular formula $C_{20}H_{32}$, and have four isoprene subunits, often known for their diverse biological effects, including anti-bacterial, anti-fungal, and anti-viral effects. Scientific reports over the past few decades, suggest that diterpenes and their derivatives can be one of the potential sources of therapeutic tools for the management of infectious diseases.

Aim: This review covers an up-to-date (2011 to July 2019) information regarding the anti-CHIKV effects of diterpenes and their derivatives on the basis of scientific evidence observed in databases.

Materials and Methods: A search was done in databases: PubMed, ScienceDirect, and Google Scholar by using relevant keywords.

Results: Findings report 121 diterpenes and their derivatives acting against CHIKV; among them, 54 were found to inhibit strongly with the EC_{50} <10 μM; while 18, 10, 10, and the rest are with 10 to <20 μM, 20 to <50 μM, 50 to <100 μM, and >100 μM, respectively.

Conclusion: More researches are necessary to investigate their possible mechanism of action behind the anti-CHIKV effect. Of note, diterpenes may be one of the important sources of anti-CHIKV drugs.

Keywords: Anti-viral drugs, Cell-based study, Chikungunya virus, Diterpenes, Diterpenoids, Terpenes.

[*] **Corresponding author Muhammad Torequl Islam:** Department of Pharmacy, Life Science Faculty, Bangabandhu Sheikh Mujibur Rahman Science and Technology University, Gopalganj (Dhaka)-8100, Bangladesh; Tel: +88026682257; Fax: +88026682173; E-mail: dmt.islam@bsmrstu.edu.bd

Anna Capasso (Ed.)

INTRODUCTION

Chikungunya virus (CHIKV), an arthropod-borne virus, causes an infectious disease characterized by fever, arthralgia and, sometimes, a maculopapular rash [1]. Unfortunately, we have no approved vaccine or antiviral treatment for CHIKV. To date, a number of compounds have been reported to act against CHIKV replication, but none have developed [2]. Therefore, the development of potent anti-CHIKV drugs is urgently needed.

Natural products from various origins are known to produce a vast array of terpenes. Among them, diterpenes containing various types of carbon skeletons (*e.g.*, jatrophane, lathyrane, myrsinane, ingenane, tigliane, daphnane, *etc.*) and their derivatives are of considerable interest due to their therapeutically relevant biological properties [3].

Diterpenes / diterpenoids are potent antioxidants; thus, these are generally protective in nature [3]. Strong antioxidants are also evident to act as pro-oxidants [4]. Therefore, these kinds of agents can be used as multi-edged like therapeutic tools [5]. On the other hand, the development of liposomal/nano-emulsion preparations manifests ease of administration of these kinds of drugs to the patients [6].

It is noteworthy that the CHIKV reached epidemic levels; therefore, the quest for novel and selective anti-CHIKV agents has been spotlighted today. This review focuses on the scientific data-based anti-CHIKV activity of diterpenes / diterpenoids and their derivatives.

SEARCH STRATEGY

An up-to-date search was made in the PubMed and ScienceDirect databases to access published articles up to July 2019. The relevant terms 'diterpenes' or 'diterpenoids' or 'derivatives of diterpenes' were paired with 'Chikungunya virus'. No language restrictions were imposed. The search yielded 68 references. Then the list was reduced to 19 references, which were further scrutinized by reading each abstract. Attention was then concentrated on 13 papers.

FINDINGS

The articles selected for this purpose is 13. An excellent review done by Remy and Litaudon (2019) listing 110 macrocyclic diterpenoids (Table **1**) acting against CHIKV, has been included in this review, along with the 12 new papers found in the databases.

Prostratin isolated from *Trigonostemon howii* was found to act against anti-CHIKV activity (EC_{50} = 2.6 μM) [7]. *Euphorbia amygdaloides* sp. derived diterpenoids were also exhibited strong anti-CHIKV activities (EC_{50}: 0.76 ± 0.14 μM) in Vero cell-based study [8].

Norcembranoids isolated from the *Sinularia kavarattiensis* at 50 and 100 μM produced moderate anti-viral activities against CHIKV [9], while 4 diterpenoids isolated from *S. lineata* showed potent to moderate anti-CHIKV activities (EC_{50}: 1.2 ± 0.2 to 11.0 ± 0.7 μM) [10]. In another study, 4'-acetoxytonantzitlolone isolated from the stem bark of *S. lineata* sp. *lineata* was also found to act against CHIKV (EC_{50}: 7 μM) [11].

Andrographolide, a bitter diterpene lactone, derived from *Andrographis paniculata* is known for its diverse biological effects, including antioxidant, anti-cancer, and anti-metabolic syndrome [12 - 14]. In a study, andrographolide (1-100 μM) was seen to act against CHKIV in HepG2 cell-based study; the EC_{50} calculated of it was 77 μM [15]. Ten jatrophane ester of *Euphorbia* extracts were seen to act against CHKIV [16], while jatrophane ester and terracinolide J isolated from the latex of *E. dendroides* exhibited anti-CHIKV activities with EC_{50} values of 5.5 ± 1.7 and 15.0 ± 3.8 μM, respectively [17]. However, 4-deoxyphorbol ester isolated from the *E. semiperfoliata* whole plant exhibited strong anti-CHIKV activity (EC_{50} = 0.45 μM) [18]. A non-oxidized lathyrane-type diterpenoid isolated from the ethyl acetate extract of the trunk bark of *Sandwithia guyanensis* showed a moderate anti-viral activity (EC_{50} = 14 μM) against CHIKV [19]. For chemical structures of some anti-CHIKV diterpenes, please see the review article done by Remy & Litaudon [20].

Diterpenes/diterpenoids and their derivatives (along with EC_{50}) acting against CHIKV have been shown in Table 1. For more information, please see the review article done by Remy & Litaudon [20].

Table 1. Diterpenes/diterpenoids and their derivatives acting against Chikungunya virus.

Diterpenes/Derivatives	Conc./Dose (Route)-Test System	EC_{50}/Effects	References
Prostratin isolated from *Trigonostemon howii*	Chikungunya virus (cell-based assay)	2.6 μM	[7]
Norcembranoids isolated from the *Sinularia kavarattiensis*	50 and 100 μM against Chikungunya virus (cell-based assay)	Moderate anti-CHIKV activities	[9]
4 diterpenoids isolated from *Stillingia lineata*	Chikungunya virus (cell-based assay)	1.2 ± 0.2 to 11.0 ± 0.7 μM	[10]

(Table 1) cont.....

Diterpenoid isolated from the *Euphorbia amygdaloides* ssp	Chikungunya virus (Vero cells)	0.76 ± 0.14 μM	[16]
Nonoxidized lathyrane-type diterpenoid isolated from the ethyl acetate extract of the trunk bark of *Sandwithia guyanensis*	Chikungunya virus (cell-based assay)	14 μM	[19]

Other diterpenes/diterpenoids and their derivatives having strong anti-CHIKV activity with EC_{50} 10 μM have been shown in Table **2**.

Table 2. Names and EC_{50}s of diterpene/diterpenoid and their derivatives acting against Chikungunya virus.

Compounds	EC_{50}s (Standard: Chloroquine 10.0 ± 5.0 μM)				
	<10	*10 to <20*	*20 to <50*	*50 to <100*	*>100*
Andrographolide				77.0 μM	
4′-acetoxytonantzitlolone	7.0 μM				
Phorbol					>343 μM
Phorbol-12-acetate					>245 μM
Phorbol-12-decanoate	4.9 ± 1.7 μM				
Phorbol-13-acetate					>174 μM
Phorbol-13-butyrate			20 ±10 μM		
Phorbol-13-decanoate	2.2 ± 0.1 μM				
Phorbol-13-tetradecanoate	0.99 ± 0.03 μM				
Phorbol-12,13-diacetate	9.4 ± 1.0 μM				
Phorbol-12,13-dibutyrate	1.8 ± 0.2 μM				
Phorbol-12,13-dihexanoate	3.2 ±0.2 μM				
Phorbol-12,13-didecanoate	6.0 ± 0.9 nM				
4-deoxyphorbol ester	0.45 μM				
4α-Phorbol-12,13-didecanoate	1.5 ± 0.1 μM				
Phorbol-13,20-diacetate			24.6 ± 7.1 μM		
Phorbol-12,13,20-triacetate			32.6 ± 4.0 μM		
12-O-Tetradecanoylphorbol-13-acetate	2.9 ± 0.3 nM				

(Table 2) cont.....

12-O-Tetradecanoyl-4α- phorbol-13-acetate	2.8 ± 0.5 μM				
12-O-Tiglylphorbol-13-decanoate	1.1 ± 0.3 μM				
12-O-(N-methylanthranilate)- phorbol-13-acetate		15.0 ± 4.0 μM			
12,13-O,O′-Dinonanoylphorbol- 20-homovanillate	0.6 ± 0.1 μM				
12-O-Phenylacetyl-13- O-acetylphorbol-20-homovanillate	1.7 ± 0.3 μM				
Trigowiin A					>100 μM
12-O-Acetylphorbol- 13(2″-methyl)-butyrate	3.3 ± 0.3 μM				
12-O-Decanoylphorbol-13-acetate	2.4 ± 0.3 μM				
12-O-Decanoyl-7-hydroperoxy- 5-ene-13-acetate phorbol	4.0 ± 0.8 μM				
20-Oxo-phorbol-12,13-dibutyrate		13.1 ± 0.5 μM			
20-Oxo-12-O-Tetradecanoylphorbol- 13-acetate	0.7 ± 0.1 μM				
12β-O-[Deca-2E,4Z-dienoyl]-13α-isobutyl- 4β-phorbol	<0.7 μM				
12β-O-[Deca-2E,4Z-dienoyl]-13α- (2-methylbutyl)-4β-phorbol	<0.7 μM				
12β-O-[Deca-2Z,4E-dienoyl]-13α- isobutyryl-4β-phorbol	<0.8 μM				
12β-O-[Deca-2Z,4E-dienoyl]-13α- isobutyryl-5-ene-7-o-o-4β-phorbol	4.5 ± 0.6 μM				
12β-O-Acetyl-4α-deoxyphorbol- 13(2″-methyl)-butyrate				77.0 μM	
12β-O-[Nona-2Z,4E,6E-trienoyl]-4α- deoxyphorbol-13-butyrate	1.4 ± 0.2 μM				
4β-Deoxyphorbol-12-tiglate-13-isobutyrate	1.0 ± 0.4 μM				
4α-Deoxyphorbol-12-tiglate-13-isobutyrate		17.0 ± 1.0 μM			
4β-Deoxyphorbol-12-acetate-13-isobutyrate	0.44 ± 0.03 μM				
12β-O-[Deca-2Z,4E-dienoyl]-13α- isobutyryl-4β-deoxyphorbol	0.9 ± 0.1 μM				
12β-O-[Deca-2Z,4E,6E-trienoyl]-13α- isobutyryl-4β-deoxyphorbol	0.6 ± 0.6 μM				
12β-O-[Octa-2Z,4E-dienoyl]-13α- isobutyryl-4β-deoxyphorbol	0.4 ± 0.02 μM				
12β-O-[Deca-2Z,4E,7Z-trienoyl]-13α- isobutyryl-4β-deoxyphorbol		12.6 ± 46.2 μM			
4α,20-Dideoxyphorbol-12-tiglate-13-isobutyrate				51.1 ± 4.1 μM	
12-Deoxyphorbol-13-acetate (prostratin)	2.7 ± 1.2 μM				

(Table 2) cont.....

3-O-Isobutyryl-12-deoxyphorbol-20-acetate	0.7 ± 0.1 μM			
13-O-Phenylacetyl-12-deoxyphorbol-20-acetate			50.8 ± 2.1 μM	
12-Deoxyphorbol-13(2"-methyl)butyrate	1.2 ± 0.2 μM			
12-Deoxyphorbol-13-[8′-oxo- hexadeca-2E,4E,6E-trienoate]	2.2 ± 1.5 μM			
12-Deoxyphorbol-13-hexadecanoate	0.02 ± 0.001 μM			
12-Deoxy-5β-hydroxy-phorbol-13-hexadecanoate	0.13 ± 0.03 μM			
12-Deoxy-6,7-epoxy-5β-hydroxy-phorbol- 13-hexadecanoate	0.09 ± 0.05 μM			
12-Deoxy-5β,6β,7α-trihydroxy-phorbol- 13-hexadecanoate	2.14 ± 0.3 μM			
4α-12-Dideoxyphorbol- 13(2,3-dimethyl)butyrate-20-acetate		>11.0 μM		
4β-12-Dideoxyphorbol- 13(2,3-dimethyl)butyrate-20-acetate	4.0 ± 0.3 μM			
Ingenol		30.1 ± 19.2 μM		
Ingenol-3-mebutate		22.9 ± 5.2 μM		
Ingenol-3,20-dibenzoate	1.2 ± 0.1 μM			
Jatrophane ester	5.5 ± 1.7 μM			
Terracinolide J		15.0 ± 3.8 μM		
Resiniferatoxin	1.8 ± 0.2 μM			
Trigocherrierin A	0.6 ± 0.1 μM			
Trigocherrin A	1.5 ± 0.6 μM			
Trigocherrin B	2.6 ± 0.7 μM			
Trigocherrin F	3.0 ± 1.2 μM			
Trigocherriolide A	1.9 ± 0.6 μM			
Trigocherriolide B	2.5 ± 0.3 μM			
Trigocherriolide C	3.9 ± 1.0 μM			

(Table 2) cont.....

Trigocherriolide E	0.7 ± 0.1 µM			
Neoguillauminin A		17.7 ± 0.8 µM		
Codiapeltine A		10.0 ± 2.3 µM		
Codiapeltine B	4.4 ± 0.5 µM			
3,5,7,8,15-Pentaacetoxy-2-hydroxy-9, 14-dioxojatropha-6(17),1-E-diene				>164.0 µM
3,5,7,15-Tetraacetoxy-2-hydroxy-8-isobutyryloxy-9, 14-dioxojatropha-6(17),11E-diene				>196.0 µM
3,5,7,15-Tetraacetoxy-2-hydroxy-8-tigloyloxy-9, 14-dioxojatroph--6(17),11E-diene	0.76 ± 0.14 µM			
3,5,7,15-Tetraacetoxy-8-benzoyloxy-2-hydroxy-9, 14-dioxojatroph--6(17),11E-diene	4.3 ± 0.2 µM			
Esulatin B			60.0 ±14.0 µM	
2,3,5,7,15- Pentaacetoxy-8-tigloyloxy-9, 14-dioxojatropha-6(17-,-11E-diene		17.4 ± 0.7 µM		
2,3,5,8,15- Pentaacetoxy-7-benzoyloxy-9, 14-dioxojatroph--6(17),11E-diene		17.1 µM		
5,7,14- Triacetoxy-3-benzoyloxy-8, 15-dihydroxy-9-oxojat--pha-6(17),11E-diene		19.5 ± 3.6 µM		
5,7-Diacetoxy-3-benzoyloxy-14, 15-dihydroxy-8-isobutyrylo-y-9-oxojatropha-6(17),11E-diene		21.0 ± 3.4 µM		
5,7-Diacetoxy-3-benzoyloxy-14, 15-dihydroxy-8-(2-methylbutyryloxy)-9-oxojatropha-6(17),11E-diene				111.0 ± 14.0 µM
5,7,14-Tri-acetoxy-3-benzoyloxy-15-hydroxy-9- oxojatropha-6(17),11E-diene			80.0 ± 6.0 µM	
Euphodendroidin E		>29.2 µM		
Euphodendroidin F			57.3 µM	
Euphodendroidin J				>144.4 µM
Euphodendroidin A		>28.6 µM		
Euphodendroidin K				>124.4 µM
Euphodendroidin L		>44.9 µM		
Euphodendroidin M		>42.8 µM		
Euphodendroidin B				133.6 µM
Euphodendroidin N		>42.5 µM		

Euphodendroidin O		27.4 µM			
Prostratin	2.6 µM				
2,3,5,7,8,9,15-Heptahydroxyjatropha-6(17), 11-diene-14-one 2,5,8, 9-tetraacetate-3-(benzoyloxyacetate)-7-(2-methyl-propionate)	5.5 ± 1.7 µM				
13α-Terracinolide G					>132.6 µM
13α-Terracinolide B					>125.6 µM
Terracinolide C		15.0 ± 3.8 µM			
Terracinolide J					>135.4 µM
3β,7β,13β, 17-O-Tetraacetyl-5α-O-benzoyl-14-oxopremyrsinol				78.0 µM	
3β,7β,15β, 17-O-Tetraacetyl-5α-O-benzoyl-14-oxopremyrsinol					>152.0 µM
3β,7β,13β, 17-O-Tetraacetyl-5α-O-(2-methylbutyryl)-1--oxopre-myrsinol			>50.0 µM		
3β,7β,13β, 17-O-Tetraacetyl-5α-O-(2-methylbutyryl)-14-oxopr--14-oxopremyrsinol					107.0 µM
7β,17-O-Diacetyl-5α-O-benzoyl-13β-nicotinyl- 3β-O-propanoyl-14-oxopremyrsinol					>107.0 µM
13β,17-O-Diacetyl-5α-O-benzoyl- 7β-hydroxy-3β-O-propano-l-14-oxopremyrsinol		11.0 ± 1.4 µM			
Premyrsinol-3-propanoate-5-benzoate-7,13,17-triacetate					>144.0 µM
5α,7β-O-Diacetyl-14β-O-benzoyl- 3β-O-propanoylmyrsinol				84.0 µM	
Tonantzitlolone A					>215.0 µM
Tonantzitlolone B		12.0 ± 3.0 µM			
Tonantzitlolone C			24.0 ± 1.0 µM		
Tonantzitlolone D					>222.0 µM
Tonantzitlolone E					>107.0 µM
Tonantzitlolone F		19.0 ± 2.0 µM			
Tonantzitlolone G					168.0 µM
Tonantzitlolone H					>191.0 µM
Tonantzitlolone I					>208.0 µM
Tonantzitloic acid					>201.0 µM

CONCLUSION AND FUTURE PERSPECTIVES

Essential oils, especially the terpenes, are one of the best candidates for treating viral infections [21]. Diterpenes, a class of chemical compounds composed of two terpene units (four isoprene units), are evident for their diverse effects, including antimicrobial, antioxidant, anti-inflammatory, and so on [22]. Diterpenes are one of the important sources of lead compounds for the development of anti-viral drugs.

In this review, among 121 diterpenes/diterpenoids and their derivatives, 54 have been found to act strongly against CHIKV (EC_{50}: <10 μM). It is evident that ngenol mebutate isolated from *Euphorbia peplus* is currently used as a topical gel (Picato®) for the treatment of keratose actinic [23]. On the other hand, tigilanol tiglate (EBC-46®) has completed safety and efficacy studies for the treatment of solid tumors in dogs [24] and is currently in a clinical study for the treatment of head and neck tumors in human adults (Link: https://qbiotics.com). However, more researches are necessary regarding the mechanism of action, and therapeutic development of diterpene-containing anti-CHIKV drugs.

CONSENT FOR PUBLICATION

Not Applicable.

CONFLICT OF INTEREST

The author declares no conflict of interest, financial or otherwise.

ACKNOWLEDGEMENTS

Declared none.

REFERENCES

[1]   Singh SK, Unni SK. Chikungunya virus: host pathogen interaction. Rev Med Virol 2011; 21(2): 78-88.
[http://dx.doi.org/10.1002/rmv.681] [PMID: 21412934]

[2]   Abdelnabi R, Neyts J, Delang L. Towards antivirals against chikungunya virus. Antiviral Res 2015; 121: 59-68.
[http://dx.doi.org/10.1016/j.antiviral.2015.06.017] [PMID: 26119058]

[3]   Islam MT, da Mata AM, de Aguiar RP, *et al.* Therapeutic potential of essential oils focusing on diterpenes. Phytother Res 2016; 30(9): 1420-44.
[http://dx.doi.org/10.1002/ptr.5652] [PMID: 27307034]

[4]   Raikos V, Neacsu M, Morrice P, Duthie G. Anti- and pro-oxidative effect of fresh and freeze-dried vegetables during storage of mayonnaise. J Food Sci Technol 2015; 52(12): 7914-23.
[http://dx.doi.org/10.1007/s13197-015-1897-x] [PMID: 26604363]

[5]   Akaberi M, Iranshahi M, Mehri S. Molecular signaling pathways behind the biological effects of

salvia species diterpenes in neuropharmacology and cardiology. Phytother Res 2016; 30(6): 878-93.
[http://dx.doi.org/10.1002/ptr.5599] [PMID: 26988179]

[6]   Islam MT. Nano-technology in aspects of phenolic drugs. British J Pharm Med Res 2017; 2(1): 306-13.

[7]   Bourjot M, Delang L, Nguyen VH, *et al.* Prostratin and 12-O-tetradecanoylphorbol 13-acetate are potent and selective inhibitors of Chikungunya virus replication. J Nat Prod 2012; 75(12): 2183-7.
[http://dx.doi.org/10.1021/np300637t] [PMID: 23215460]

[8]   Nothias-Scaglia LF, Retailleau P, Paolini J, *et al.* Jatrophane diterpenes as inhibitors of *chikungunya virus* replication: structure-activity relationship and discovery of a potent lead. J Nat Prod 2014; 77(6): 1505-12.
[http://dx.doi.org/10.1021/np500271u] [PMID: 24926807]

[9]   Lillsunde KE, Festa C, Adel H, *et al.* Bioactive cembrane derivatives from the Indian Ocean soft coral, *Sinularia kavarattiensis.* Mar Drugs 2014; 12(7): 4045-68.
[http://dx.doi.org/10.3390/md12074045] [PMID: 25056629]

[10]   Olivon F, Palenzuela H, Girard-Valenciennes E, *et al.* Antiviral Activity of Flexibilane and Tigliane Diterpenoids from *Stillingia lineata.* J Nat Prod 2015; 78(5): 1119-28.
[http://dx.doi.org/10.1021/acs.jnatprod.5b00116] [PMID: 25946116]

[11]   Techer S, Girard-Valenciennes E, Retailleau P, *et al.* Tonantzitlolones from *Stillingia lineata* ssp. *lineata* as potential inhibitors of chikungunya virus. Phytochem Lett 2015; 12: 313-9.
[http://dx.doi.org/10.1016/j.phytol.2015.04.023]

[12]   Islam MT. Andrographolide, an up-coming multi-edged plant-derived sword in cancers. Asian J ethnopharmacol med foods 2016; 2(5): 1-3.

[13]   Islam MT. Andrographolide, a new hope in the prevention and treatment of metabolic syndrome. Front Pharmacol 2017; 8: 571.
[http://dx.doi.org/10.3389/fphar.2017.00571] [PMID: 28878680]

[14]   Islam MT, Ali ES, Uddin SJ, *et al.* Andrographolide, a diterpene lactone from *Andrographis paniculata* and its therapeutic promises in cancer. Cancer Lett 2018; 420(420): 129-45.
[http://dx.doi.org/10.1016/j.canlet.2018.01.074] [PMID: 29408515]

[15]   Wintachai P, Kaur P, Lee RC, *et al.* Activity of andrographolide against chikungunya virus infection. Sci Rep 2015; 5: 14179.
[http://dx.doi.org/10.1038/srep14179] [PMID: 26384169]

[16]   Nothias-Scaglia LF, Schmitz-Afonso I, Renucci F, *et al.* Insights on profiling of phorbol, deoxyphorbol, ingenol and jatrophane diterpene esters by high performance liquid chromatography coupled to multiple stage mass spectrometry. J Chromatogr A 2015; 1422: 128-39.
[http://dx.doi.org/10.1016/j.chroma.2015.09.092] [PMID: 26522744]

[17]   Esposito M, Nothias LF, Nedev H, *et al.* *Euphorbia dendroides* latex as a source of jatrophane esters: isolation, structural analysis, conformational study, and anti-chikv activity. J Nat Prod 2016; 79(11): 2873-82.
[http://dx.doi.org/10.1021/acs.jnatprod.6b00644] [PMID: 27786472]

[18]   Nothias LF, Boutet-Mercey S, Cachet X, *et al.* Environmentally friendly procedure based on supercritical fluid chromatography and tandem mass spectrometry molecular networking for the discovery of potent antiviral compounds from *Euphorbia semiperfoliata.* J Nat Prod 2017; 80(10): 2620-9.
[http://dx.doi.org/10.1021/acs.jnatprod.7b00113] [PMID: 28925702]

[19]   Remy S, Olivon F, Desrat S, *et al.* Structurally diverse diterpenoids from *Sandwithia guyanensis.* J Nat Prod 2018; 81(4): 901-12.
[http://dx.doi.org/10.1021/acs.jnatprod.7b01025] [PMID: 29493237]

[20]   Remy S, Litaudon M. Macrocyclic diterpenoids from euphorbiaceae as a source of potent and selective

inhibitors of chikungunya virus replication. Molecules 2019; 24(12): E2336.
[http://dx.doi.org/10.3390/molecules24122336] [PMID: 31242603]

[21]   Schnitzler P. Essential oils for the treatment of herpes simplex virus infections. Chemotherapy 2019; 64(1): 1-7.
[http://dx.doi.org/10.1159/000501062] [PMID: 31234166]

[22]   Aminimoghadamfarouj N, Nematollahi A. Propolis Diterpenes as a Remarkable Bio-Source for Drug Discovery Development: A Review. Int J Mol Sci 2017; 18(6): E1290.
[http://dx.doi.org/10.3390/ijms18061290] [PMID: 28629133]

[23]   Rosen RH, Gupta AK, Tyring SK. Dual mechanism of action of ingenol mebutate gel for topical treatment of actinic keratoses: rapid lesion necrosis followed by lesion-specific immune response. J Am Acad Dermatol 2012; 66(3): 486-93.
[http://dx.doi.org/10.1016/j.jaad.2010.12.038] [PMID: 22055282]

[24]   Miller J, Campbell J, Blum A, *et al.* Dose characterization of the investigational anticancer drug tigilanol tiglate (EBC-46) in the local treatment of canine mast cell tumors. Front Vet Sci 2019; 6: 106.
[http://dx.doi.org/10.3389/fvets.2019.00106] [PMID: 31111038]

CHAPTER 6

Design Development and Evaluation of Anti-Inflammatory Nanogel For The Treatment of Psoriasis

A.A. Yelmate[*], P. Gundewar and **R.S. Moon**

School of Pharmacy, S.R.T.M. University, Nanded, Maharashtra, India

Abstract: Psoriasis is an anti-inflammatory condition associated with painful, itchy skin and typical skin lesions. Usually, psoriasis is characterized by the appearance of thick, red, scaly patches on the skin and build-up of dead skin cells leading to painful inflammation in the joints. Due to the lack of possible cure and the disadvantages of allopathic medicines, there is a need to develop new formulations from natural products having antipsoriatic activity. *Argemone Mexicana* Linn. acts as an anti-inflammatory drug for the treatment of psoriasis with no side effects as compared to synthetic drugs. Considering the anti-inflammatory activity, the attempt was made to develop a new herbal formulation for anti-inflammatory study. The developed formulations were subjected to physicochemical evaluation.

Keywords: *Argemone Mexicana* Linn, Inflammation, Nanogel, Oedema, Psoriasis.

INTRODUCTION

Argemone mexicana L, known as pila datura, belonging to family Papaveraceae, is a common weed widely distributed in many tropical and sub-tropical countries [1]. It is a herb commonly known as prickly poppy or Mexican poppy and is found everywhere in India [2]. Mexicana linn. is known as kaju and Ahon ekun. A. mexicana is considered to be one of the important medicinal plants from India. Its juice is yellow in colour which exudes when the plant is broken or injured; it is used in India as a traditional medicine for the treatment of different ailments like dropsy, jaundice and a number of cutaneous infections. Different parts like root, seed, leaves, flowers of the plant are used in the treatment of chronic skin diseases and used as an emetic, expectorant, demulcent and diuretic, *etc*. The seeds oil is used as a remedy for the treatment of a number of intestinal infections [3, 4].

[*] **Corresponding author A.A. Yelmate:** School of Pharmacy, S.R.T.M. University, Nanded, Maharashtra, India; Tel: 0982 233 6268; E-mail: archanayelmate1@gmail.com

Anna Capasso (Ed.)

Its leaves and seeds are also responsible for maintaining normal blood circulation as well as cholesterol levels in the human body [5]. The infusion made from this plant is used in hypertension [6].

MATERIALS AND METHODS

Collection of Plant Material

The plant materials for the study included leaves and stems of *A. Mexicana.* The plant materials were collected from Latur Dist. Maharashtra in Oct-Nov and the plant materials were taxonomically authenticated by Dr. Mullani, School of life science, SRTM University Nanded, Maharashtra.

Extraction of Plant Material

Fresh plant materials (leaves and stems) of *argemone mexicana* linn were collected from the local region of the Latur district. Collected plant materials were washed under running tap water in order to remove adhering dust and other earthy matter, dried under shade and the coarse powder was prepared in a mechanical grinder. The coarse powder was extracted successively with each of the solvents with varying polarity, namely water, N-butanol and methanol, by maceration for 48 hours. The crude extract was filtered using the Whatmann filter paper and solvents were evaporated to dryness by using a water bath. Finally, dried extract was stored in a refrigerator and used for further study [7, 8].

FORMULATIONS OF NANOGEL

Preparation of Drug-Loaded Nanodispersions

Nano dispersion of the drug was prepared by the modified emulsification-diffusion method. In this method, 100 mg of the drug (extract) was weighed and dissolved in 10 ml of 10% DMSO containing tween. This was the organic phase containing drug-polymer mixture. This phase was added slowly into a 30 ml aqueous phase containing sodium alginate with constant stirring at 1000-2000 rpm using a magnetic stirrer. The addition of organic phase directly into the aqueous solution was done carefully with the help of a syringe with a needle. At this stage, the solution was stirred for at least 6 min at a continuous speed. Then distilled water was added slowly to the solution with stirring for 1 hour for the diffusion of an organic layer in the continuous phase, leading to the formation of nanodispersion [9].

Preparation of Nanogel

Gels of the nanodispersion were prepared by dispersing a gelling agent (carbopol 940) in the nanodispersion of the drug) by using a high-speed stirrer. The pH was adjusted to 7.0 by using a surfactant to form the gel, and *argemone mexicana* linn leaves and seed extract with gels were stored at room temperature [10].

Formulation Batches of Nanogel

Table 1. Formulation Composition.

Ingredients	Batches			
	F1	**F2**	**F3**	**F4**
Drug extract	1% (aqueous)	1% (aqueous)	1% (methanolic)	1% (methanolic)
Sodium alginate	1%	2%	2%	1%
Tween	0.5 ml	0.5 ml	0.5 ml	0.5 ml
Carbopol 940	2%	1%	1%	2%
BHT	0.2%	0.2%	0.2%	0.2%
Propyl paraben	0.4%	0.4%	0.4%	0.4%
Distilled water	50 ml	50 ml	50 ml	50 ml

EVALUATION OF DEVELOPED FORMULATION

Appearance

All developed nanogel formulations were evaluated for homogeneity, presence of any foreign particles, and colour by visual inspection after the gels have been filled in the final container for storage.

Determination of pH

The pH of all the developed nanogels was determined using a digital pH meter. The readings were taken for an average of 3 times. The results are shown in Table 1.

Determination of Homogeneity

All developed nanogels were tested for homogeneity; the uniformity was evaluated by visual inspection after the gels have been filled in the final container. They were tested for their appearance and presence of any foreign particles and aggregates. All selected formulation batches were tested and good results were obtained in the homogeneity test.

Viscosity

Viscosities of the all developed nanogels were measured with the help of Brookfield viscometer.

Particle Size

The mean size of all selected herbal nanogels was determined by using Malvern Mastersizer 2000 MS (Malvern Instruments UK).

Spreadability

The spreadability of all formulations was determined by an apparatus suggested by Multimer *et al.*, which was fabricated in the laboratory and used for this study. This apparatus consists of a wooden block, which is fixed with a glass slide and movable glass slide, and its one end is tied to a weight pan rolled on the pulley.

Skin Irritancy Test

Skin irritancy test was performed on healthy human skin. Nanogel was applied on the arm twice daily at an interval of 12 h, and the skin was monitored for development of rashes or irritations after the subsequent application of nanogel for 72 h. No allergic symptoms like inflammation, redness, swelling, irritations appeared on the healthy human skin. Hence the prepared nanogel formulation was found to be stable and free from skin irritation on application to healthy human skin [11].

RESULTS AND DISCUSSION

pH: The pH values of all developed formulations were in the range of 6-7, which is considered acceptable to avoid irritation upon application to the skin. The pH of the various gel formulations was determined by using a digital pH meter. pH was found to be well within the limits of skin pH, *i.e.* 5.6-7.5. Hence it was concluded that all the formulations did not cause any local irritation to the skin (Table **2**).

Particle Size Determination

All the prepared nanogels showed a mean particle size ranging from 253-442 nm after their dilutions in distilled water, which was well within the limits (Table **3**).

Table 2. Physicochemical evaluation of formulations.

Batches	pH	Homogeneity	Viscosity	Spreadability	Irritancy Test
F1	7.1	Fair	65,240.06	10.25	N
F2	6.4	Good	92,467.03	10.75	N
F3	6.8	Good	1,24,000.01	10.70	N
F4	6.0	Good	1,40,647.30	11.75	N

N= sign of no irritation

Table 3. Results of Particle Size Distribution.

Formulation Batches	Particle Size (Nm)
F1	442
F2	270
F3	253
F4	285

Zeta Potential Measurements

Stability Studies

Optimized formulation (f3) was subjected to stability studies. Various parameters such as pH, viscosity, homogeneity, consistency, and appearance were evaluated after 0, 30, 60 days of stability. The results of the stability studies are shown in the following table; the result shows that there is no significant change in the evaluated parameters during stability studies. Thus it can be proved from the stability studies that the prepared formulation is stable and not much affected by elevated temperature condition (Table **4**).

Table 4. Results of stability study.

Time (days)	pH	Homogeneity	Viscosity	Spreadability
0	6.8	Good	1,40,647.30	10.25
30	6.6	Good	1,40,647.15	10.24
60	6.4	Good	1,40,647.20	10.20
90	6.4	Good	1,40,647.25	10.21

HORIBA- SZ100Z

Measurement Results

Date	: Tuesday, March 13, 2007 10:47:15 PM
Measurement Type	: Zeta Potential
Sample Name	: 04/03/15 viky
Temperature of the Holder	: 25.1 °C
Dispersion Medium Viscosity	: 0.893 mPa·s
Conductivity	: 0.196 mS/cm
Electrode Voltage	: 3.3 V

Calculation Results

Peak No.	Zeta Potential	Electrophoretic Mobility
1	-24.0 mV	-0.000186 cm2/Vs
2	--- mV	--- cm2/Vs
3	--- mV	--- cm2/Vs

Zeta Potential (Mean)   : -24.0 mV
Electrophoretic Mobility Mean : -0.000186 cm2/Vs

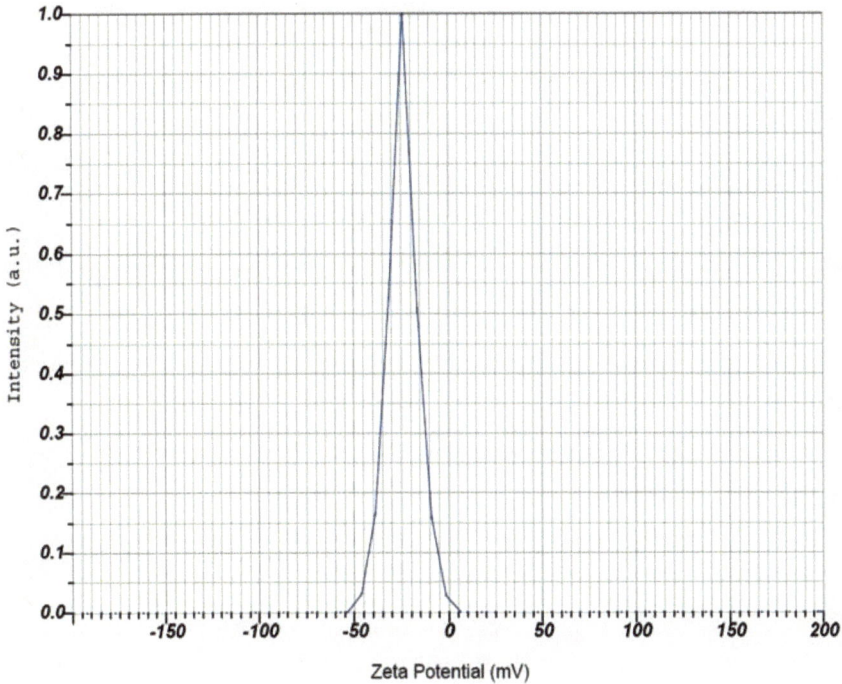

IN-VIVO ANTI-INFLAMMATORY ACTIVITY

Animals

For this study, healthy Wistar albino mice (20-30 g) of either sex and of the same age were used. They were individually kept under standard environmental conditions and maintained in clean cages and fed with commercially pellet diet (M/s Hindustan Lever Ltd., Mumbai) and water *ad libitum*. The experimental protocols for the study were approved by the Institutional Animal Ethics Committee for experimental clearance (No. 1613/PO/a/12/CPCSEA). For the study, all animal procedures were followed in the three groups (Control, Test and Standard) with six animals each [12, 13].

Carrageenan-Induced Mice Paw Oedema Method

Animals were made to fast for 24 hrs before the experiment with water *ad libitum*. Approximately, 50uL of 1% suspension of carrageenan in saline was prepared 1 h before each experiment and injected into the plantar side of the right hind paw of mice. 0.2 g of herbal gel containing 1% *A.Mexicana* extract was applied to the plantar surface of the hind paw by slowly rubbing for two to three times with the index finger. In mice of the control groups, only plain gel base was applied and 0.2 g 1% Diclofenac gel was applied in the standard group. Formulations without extract were applied 1h before the carrageenan injection. Group I was recognized as (negative control) carrageenan (0.1 ML of 1% carrageenan/mouse to the sub plantar region and saline water 0.1 ML/kg bw). Group II was recognized as (positive control) carrageenan + Diclofenac Gel *(2.5 mg/kg BW)*. Group III was recognized as (treated group) carrageenan + Gel of *Argemone Mexicana containing Methanolic extract (0.2g/kg BW)*. Group IV was recognized as (treated group) carrageenan + Gel of *Argemone Mexicana containing Aqueous extract (0.2g/kg BW)*.

The paw volume was measured at an interval of half an hour after carrageenan injection, using Plethysmometer (orchid scientific and innovative pvt). The left hind paw was observed as a reference and the non-inflamed paw for comparison. The average percentage increase in paw volume with the time was calculated and compared against the control group [14].

Statistical Analysis

Data from the studies were reported as the mean ± S.E.M. and analyzed statistically by means of the analysis of variance (ANOVA) followed by Student t-test. Values of $*p<0.05$ were considered as significant.

RESULTS AND DISCUSSION

Table 5. Effect of topical administration of Herbal gel on carrageenan-induced mice paw oedema.

Time (min)	Treatment			
	Negative	**Positive**	**Methanolic**	**Aqueous**
0 min	0.107±0.013	0.107±0.013	0.102±0.015	0.11±0.021
30 min	0.167±0.015	0.107±0.014	0.14±0.015*	0.15±0.015
60 min	0.217±0.019	0.164±0.009**	0.17±0.013**	0.204±0.013
120 min	0.255±0.013	0.19±0.011**	0.205±0.014**	0.245±0.013
180 min	0.279±0.010	0.219±0.010**	0.232±0.015**	0.267±0.011

DISCUSSION AND CONCLUSION

Psoriasis is mainly characterized by T-cell activation that releases pro-inflammatory cytokines such as TNF-α factor, which leads to keratinocyte proliferation, forming the skin lesions. The major manifestation of psoriasis is a chronic inflammation of the skin. During an active state of this disease, an underlying inflammatory mechanism is frequently involved. The present work formulated a novel herbal nanogel using *Argemone mexicana linn.* Its leaves and stem extract possess a better anti-inflammatory activity with good consistency and stability properties. In this work, an attempt has been made to treat psoriasis by using natural remedies having the power to treat the underlying cause of inflammation.

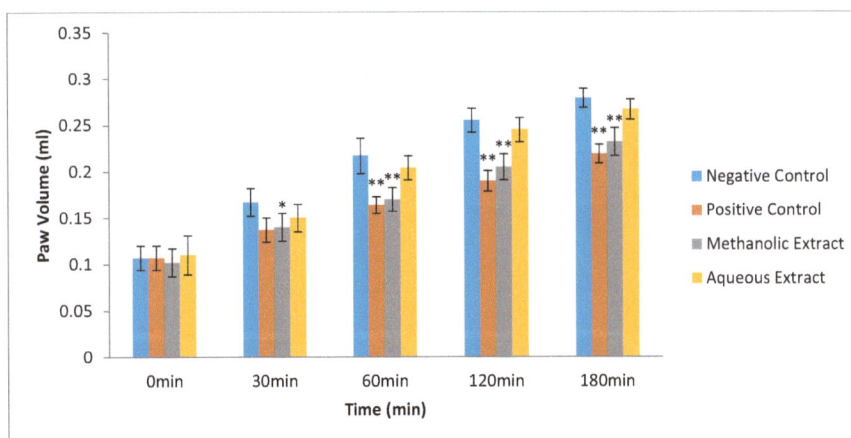

Fig. (1). Topical administration of Herbal gel on carrageenan-induced mice paw oedema.

The anti-inflammatory activity after topical application of herbal nanogel formulations was studied. Carrageenan-induced hind paw oedema is the standard experimental model of acute inflammation. Moreover, the experimental model exhibits a high degree of reproducibility. Carrageenan induced oedema is a biphasic response. The first phase is mediated through the release of inflammatory cytokines like histamine, serotonin and kinins, whereas the second phase is related to the release of prostaglandin and slow reacting substances. The results of anti-inflammatory activity after topical administration of herbal gel are reported in Table **5** and Fig. **1**. Statistical analysis showed that the oedema inhibition by prepared nanodispersion containing methanolic extract significantly differed from the control group. The results showed that the anti-inflammatory effect of the formulation containing 1% of the herbal gel of methanolic extract was better than aqueous extract and the effect of formulation containing methanolic extract was equivalent to the effect of standard gel formulation. From these overall results, we can conclude that topical preparation containing 1% of methanolic extract of *argemone mexicana linn* possessed anti-inflammatory activity similar to the formulation containing aqueous extract; this effect can be useful for the treatment of local inflammation. The initial physicochemical parameters of formulations, *i.e.* pH, viscosity, particle size and stability were also examined. The pH of all formulations was near to about 6.8, being in the normal range of the skin. The preparation was stable under normal storage conditions and did not produce any skin irritation, *i.e.* erythema and edema for about a month when applied over the skin.

CONSENT FOR PUBLICATION

Not Applicable.

CONFLICT OF INTEREST

The author declares no conflict of interest, financial or otherwise.

ACKNOWLEDGEMENTS

Declared none.

REFERENCES

[1]   Sourabie TS, Nikiema JB, Nacoulma OG, *et al.* Monographycal survey of pharmacological potentials of *Argemone mexicana* L. (papaveraceae), a plant of burkina faso pharmacopeia: *Determination of antihepatotoxic and antipyretic activities.* IJRBS 2014; 1(2): 1-10.

[2]   Chetna G, Munish A, Surendra KS, *et al.* preparation and evaluation of anti-inflammatory activity of gugulipid-loaded proniosomal gel. acta Poloniae Pharmaceutica n. Drug Res 2011; 689(1): 147-50.

[3]   Bhalke RD, Gosavi SA. Anti-stress and antiallergic effect of *Argemone mexicana* stems in asthma. Arch Pharm Sci Res 2009; 1: 127-9.

[4]   de Albuquerque UP, Monteiro JM, Ramos MA, de Amorim EL. Medicinal and magic plants from a public market in northeastern Brazil. J Ethnopharmacol 2007; 110(1): 76-91. [http://dx.doi.org/10.1016/j.jep.2006.09.010] [PMID: 17056216]

[5]   Minu V, Harsh V, Ravikant T, Paridhi J, Noopur S. Medicinal plants of Chhattisgarh with anti-snake venom property. Int J Curr Pharm Rev Res 2012; 3: 1-10.

[6]   Brahmachari G, Gorai D, Roy R. Review: *Argemone mexicana*: chemical and pharmacological aspects. Rev bras farmacogn 2013; 23(3): 559-75.

[7]   Prakash PR, Rao NGR, Soujanya C. Formulation evaluation and anti-inflammatory activity of topical Etoricoxib gel. Asian J Pharm Clin Res 2010; 3(2): 126-9.

[8]   Brain KR, Turner TD. The practical evaluation of phytopharmaceauticals. Bristol: wright-scientia 1975; pp. 57-8.

[9]   Sofowara A. Medicinal plants and traditional medicine in Africa. Ibadan: spectrum books 1993; pp. 151-3.

[10]   Veni T, Pushpanathan T. Investigation of Antimicrobial and phytochemical analysis of *Argemone mexicana* medicinal plants extracts against bacteria with gastrointestinal relevance. Asian J Pharm Clin Res 2014; 7(2): 93-7.

[11]   Sultana F, Manirujjaman , Imran-Ul-Haque M, Arafat M, Sharmin S. An overview of nanogel drug delivery system. J Appl Pharm Sci 2013; 3(8): s95-s105.

[12]   Phatak Atul A, Chaudhari Praveen D. Development and evaluation of nanogel as a carrier for transdermal delivery of aceclofenac. Asian J Pharm Tech 2012; 2(4): 125-32.

[13]   Osho A, Adetunji T. Antimicrobial activity of the essential oil of *Argemone Mexicana* Linn. J Med Plant Res 2010; 4(1): 19-22.

[14]   Ibrahim HA, Ibrahim H. Phytochemical screening and toxicity evaluation on the leaves of *Argemone Mexicana* Linn (Papaveraceae). Int J App Sci 2009; 3: pp. 39-43.

CHAPTER 7

Antilithiatic Properties of Moroccan Medicinal Plants and Mechanism Insights of their Phytochemicals

Aya Khouchlaa*, **Abdelhakim Bouyahya** and **M'hamed Tijane**

Department of Biology, Faculty of Science, Genomic Center of Human Pathologies, Faculty of Medicine, Laboratory of Human Pathologies Biology, Mohammed V University, Rabat, Morocco

Abstract: The transition from raw herbs to synthetic pharmaceuticals bioactive compounds has undergone evolution and herbal medicine has become an important source of raw materials to treat different illnesses. Indeed, the alternative treatment using herbal medicine has come into demand in recent years and has renewed interest in the plants that are effective, safe, and culturally acceptable. In Morocco, several medicinal plants are used traditionally to treat kidney stones and *in vitro* and *in vivo* experimental studies have proved their antilithiasic activity. This review aims to list all *in vitro* and *in vivo* antilithiasic medicinal plants used by the Moroccan population and to present bioactive compounds responsible for this activity. Further, we determined some molecular targets by these bioactive compounds.

Keywords: Crystallization, Kidney stones, Phyto-molecules, Urinary.

INTRODUCTION

Herbal medicine comes from the Greek word "phyto" meaning plant and "therapeuein" meaning cure [1]. Since ancient times, a series of failures and successes have been encountered in using medicinal plants for healing, pain relief, cure headaches, and heal wounds [2]. From generation to generation, the humans have passed on their knowledge and experience whose main objective was based on the idea to overcome suffering and improve their health [3].

Parts of plants used in herbal medicine produce a large number of active substances. The diversity of these substances and the fact that they are not found in all plants show that they do not involve general metabolism. So, they are known as secondary metabolites [4]. These latter comprise generally two types of

---

* Corresponding author Aya Khouchlaa: Department of Biology, Faculty of Science, Genomic Center of Human Pathologies, Faculty of Medicine, Laboratory of Human Pathologies Biology, Mohammed V University, Rabat, Morocco; Tel: 00212674158222; E-mail: aya.khouchlaa@gmail.com

Anna Capasso (Ed.)

compounds. Phenolic compounds take part in plant-plant interactions (allelopathic inhibition of germination and growth) [5] and the nitrogen compounds include alkaloids and glycosides. The latter release out hydrocyanic acid when the plants are damaged. They are synthesized from amino acids. These metabolites often play a defensive role in the plant which they manufacture [5].

A variety of structurally secondary metabolites are produced as a means for plants to defend themselves against herbivores, bacteria, fungi, and viruses. The secondary metabolites represent an exciting library of bioactive compounds filtered by natural selection, which have been used by humans to treat infections and health disorders, or as spices and perfumes [4]. Many medicinal plants have been used around the world to fight against several illnesses such as microbial diseases, metabolic disorders, and other human complications [6-9]. Numerous empirical studies using several ethnomedicinal approaches have demonstrated the efficacy of medicinal plants as a remedy against kidney illness [10-13]. Phytochemical screening is one of the techniques to identify new sources of therapeutically and industrially important compounds present in the plant extracts to treat a specific disease [14].

In this review, the antilithiasic properties of Moroccan medicinal plants have been reported. The mechanism insights of some phytochemicals against lithiasis were discussed in this review.

METHODS

The current review was done on the research of the scientific data published regarding experimental medicinal plants use against urolithiasis. The researches were obtained using various databases, including PubMed, Springer, Science Direct, Scopus, Google Scholar, Hindawi, and Taylor & Francis.

RESULTS AND DISCUSSION

Ethnobotany of Antilithiasic Medicinal Plants Used in Morocco

Ethnobotany is a discipline that reflects the relationship between human and their habitat for the purpose to search solutions against illnesses. Morocco presents a key reservoir of medicinal plants for traditional use to treat several pathologies, including urinary lithiasis. Numerous studies identifying antilithiasic plants have been reported based on ethnobotanical approaches [15 - 24].

Various traditional uses of medicinal plants have been reported in different areas of Morocco. In the Tan-Tan region, located in sub-Mediterranean bioclimatic Sahara with a temperate winter climate, Ghourri *et al.* identified 50 species with a predominant *Apiaceae* family: *Ammi visnaga, Ammodaucus leucotrichus, Apium graveolens, Daucus carotta, Eryngium triquetrum, Foeniculum vulgare,* and *Petroselinum sativum.* Among the use of medicinal species, the leaves and seeds have been widely used as a decoction to treat nephrolithiasis [15]. Similar plants have been reported by El Hafiane *et al.* in an ethnobotanical study conducted in the South of Morocco (Agadir). This study showed the use of *Ammi visnaga, Crocus sativus, Cynodon dactylon,* and *Petroselinum sativum* to treat kidney stones [20].

An ethnobotanical study conducted by Khouchlaa *et al.* in Western Morocco (Rabat) mentioned 35 species with a predominant *Caryophylaceae* family. The most cited plant of this family was *Herniaria hirsuta.* The Arabic vernacular name of this plant was "Harasset lahjar", which means "stones dissolution" [18]. Some medicinal plants reported in this study have not been mentioned in the study conducted in the Sahara region, such as *Aloe vera, Anthemis nobilis, Taraxacum officinalis, Caralluma europaea, Saccharum officinarum,* and *Prunus cerasus.* From this perspective, it is important to extend other ethnopharmacological studies in various Moroccan regions in order to identify all medicinal plants used for the treatment of lithiasis and safeguard the knowledge of the Moroccan population.

Other Moroccan ethnobotanical studies reported the use of medicinal plants against different diseases such as diabetes, cancer, allergy, respiratory affection, and urolithiasis. From these researches, we observed a few medicinal plants reported against urolithiasis. *Allium sativum* and *Origanum vulgare* have been reported in the north-central region of Morocco (Fès) [16]. In Settat, four plants used in the treatment of kidney stones have been cited: *Artemisia absinthium, Lavandula dentate, Zea mays, and Petroselinum sativum* [24]. In the North West of Morocco (Kenitra), *Ammi visnaga, Herniaria hirsuta,* Vicia faba, Lavandula dentate, and *Rosmarinus officinalis* have been reported [17 - 25]. In this context, further specific ethnobotanical studies on antilithiasis plants should be conducted in other Moroccan regions to identify all medicinal plants used traditionally to treat lithiasis. These perspectives can open a way for their pharmacological studies and the identification of bioactive molecules that could treat or/and prevent kidney stones.

Experimental Methods to Evaluate The Antilithiatic Activity

In Vitro Methods

The antilithiatic effects of Moroccan medicinal plants have been extensively studied using various experimental approaches. Table **1** summarizes several *in vitro* methods used to reveal the effects of plant extracts against stone formation. Several *in vitro* assays have been used by authors to prove the effect of organic and aqueous extracts of medicinal plants, such as the litholytic effect and crystallization of calcium oxalate (CaOx) in synthetic and human urine.

Table 1. Antilithiatic effect of different Moroccan medicinal plant extracts.

Species (family) Reported in Moroccan Ethnobotanical Studies	Part Used	Extracts	Method Used	Outcome	Ref
Allium sativum (Liliaceae) [15 - 16]	Bulbs	Ethanol, petroleum ether, aqueous extract	*In vitro* titrimetric assay	33.9%, 26.9%, 13.2% of calcium inhibition; respectively	[44]
Ammi visnaga (Apiaceae) [15 - 17]	Fruit	aqueous extract	*In vitro* cultured renal epithelial cells assays	Injured LLC-PK1 and MDCK cells when exposed to Ox	[45]
	Seed	aqueous extract	*In vitro* litholytic effect on cystine urinary calculi	Complete and quick dissolution of cystine urinary calculi	[10]
			In vivo oxaluria induced by glycolic acid added to the diet for 4 weeks	Decreased urinary supersaturating in salts promoter of oxalocalcic lithiasis by a diuretic effect.	[40]
			In vivo human urinary test	Expulsion of stones through urine from kidney and urethras	[46]
Atriplex halimus (Chenopodiaceae) [15]	Leaves	aqueous extract	*In vitro* oxalate crystallization in synthetic urine	68.79% inhibitory effects of 50% physiological concentrations of plant extract on oxalate crystallisation	[47]

Species (family) Reported in Moroccan Ethnobotanical Studies	Part Used	Extracts	Method Used	Outcome	Ref
Citrus limon (Rutaceae) [15 - 19]	Fruit	Juice	*In vitro* turbidimetric method on calcium oxalate crystallization *In vivo* inhibitory effect in human urine	A significant dose dependent reducing rate of calcium oxalate in *in vitro* assays. Increase in urinary pH (from 6.7 to 6.9) and increased excretion of oxalate calcium and citrate with 33. 41% and 6. 85 % respectively in *in vivo* assays.	[30]
	Peel	n-hexane, chloroform, and ethanol extract	*In vivo* oxaluric acid induced by ethylene glycol in rats.	Significantly higher urinary calcium and oxalate excretion (4.47 and 18.86mg/24 h, respectively)	[48]
Crocus sativus L. *(Iridaceae)* [15 - 20 - 21]	Stigmates of the flower	Aqueous extract	*In vivo* ethylene glycol induced nephrolithiasis in rats	- Reduced MDA levels (a lipid peroxidation product) in prophylactic and curative treatment - Protected against ethylene glycol induced calcium oxalate (CaOx) nephrolithiasis	[32]
Cynodon dactylon (Poaceae) [15 - 21]	Roots	hydroalcoholic extract	*In vivo* ethylene glycol induced nephrolithiasis in rats	- The number of deposits was significantly lower compared with no treated group - Decreased the weight of stones - Urine oxalate level decreased in nephrolithiasis rats treated with the extract	[49]
	nd	Aqueous extract	*In vitro* calcium oxalate crystallization	Presents an inhibiting effect of a rate of 20 % on the crystalline growth and 60 % on the phase of aggregation	[50]

(Table 1) cont.....

Species (family) Reported in Moroccan Ethnobotanical Studies	Part Used	Extracts	Method Used	Outcome	Ref
Herniaria hirsuta (Caryophyllaceae) [15-17-22]	Whole plant	Aqueous extract	*In vitro* calcium oxalate crystallization in human urine	- Promoted the nucleation of calcium oxalate crystals, increasing their number but decreasing their size; - Favored the formation of calcium oxalate dehydrates rather than monohydrate crystals.	[51]
	Whole plant	Aqueous extract	*In vivo* calcium oxalate stones induced by ethylene glycol in rats	- Higher magnesium content in nephrolithic rats; - Crystalluria was characterized by the excretion of smaller crystals in nephrolithic rats; - The histology showed no deposits of CaOx crystals in those of treated rats.	[36 - 37]
	Whole plant	Aqueous extract	*In vitro* litholytic effect on cystine urinary calculi	Complete dissolution of cystine urinary calculi	[10]
Hordeum vulgare (Poaceae) [15]	Seed	Aqueous extract	*In vitro* turbidimetric method on calcium oxalate crystallization	A very slight inhibition (6%) of crystallization of calcium oxalate monohydrate by reducing their size	[31]
		Ethanolic extract	*In vivo* calcium oxalate placed in renal Wistar albino rats	Increased renal calcium oxalate excretion	[52]
Opuntia ficus-indica (Cactaceae) [15 - 21]	Flowers	aqueous extract	*In vitro* litholytic effect on cystine urinary calculi	Complete dissolution of cystine urinary calculi	[10]

(Table 1) cont.....

Species (family) Reported in Moroccan Ethnobotanical Studies	Part Used	Extracts	Method Used	Outcome	Ref
Petroselinum sativum (Apiaceae) [15 - 19 - 20 - 23 - 24]	nd	Aqueous extract	*In vivo* renal calculi induced by ethylene glycol in male albino rats	- Restored the urine pH to normal and significantly increased the urine volume and magnesium; - Increased lipid peroxidation in the kidneys in the lithogenic treatment; - Microscopic and histopathological examinations revealed an inhibition of renal stone associated with a decrease in calcium kidney content in prophylactic and curative treatment.	[38]
	Aerial parts		*In vivo* ethylene glycol-induced kidney calculi in rats.	Reduced the growth of urinary stones and hepatotoxicity induction by ethylene glycol in rats	[39]
Raphanus sativus (Brassicaceae) [18]		Juice	Measurement of human urinary pH	Effects were not proved	[53]
	Leaves	Methanolic extract	*In vivo* urolithiasis induced by ethylene glycol and ammonium chloride in rats	Inhibited significantly the formation of kidney stones	[54]
Saccharum spontaneum Linn. *(Poaceae)* [18]	Root	Ethanolic extract	*In vivo* ethylene glycol induced lithiasis in rats	Reduced level of β--glucuronidasein, n-acetyl-d-glucosaminidase, and xanthine oxidase	[35]

(Table 1) cont.....

Species (family) Reported in Moroccan Ethnobotanical Studies	Part Used	Extracts	Method Used	Outcome	Ref
Zea mays (Poaceae) [15 - 24]	Corn silk	Aqueous extract	*In vivo* urinary risk factors with specific diet	The extract did not influence citraturia, calciuria or urinary pH values.	[55]
			In vitro litholytic effect on cystine urinary calculi	Complete and quick dissolution of cystine urinary calculi	[10]
			In vivo diuretic effect in Wistar male rats	No significant diuresis result, but the combination with *Tribulus terrestris* extracts have a diuretic effect accompanied by increased sodium, potassium and urinary chlorine levels	[43]
Zingiber Officinale (Zingiberaceae) [18]	Rhizomes	Ethanolic extract	*In vivo* ethylene glycol-induced urolithiasis in rats	- Significantly increased urine output - Significantly reduced urinary excretion of calcium, phosphate, uric acid, magnesium, and urea. - significantly lowered deposition of stone in kidneys of calculogenic rats by curative and preventive treatment	[33]
Zizyphus lotus (Rhamnaceae) [15-18-21-22]	Fruit	Aqueous extract	*In vitro* litholytic effect on calcium oxalate and urate urinary calculi	Important dissolution on urate urinary calculi than calcium oxalate	[13]
			In vitro oxalate crystallization in human urine	Decreased the size and number of calcium oxalate crystals at 10 mg/mL	[55]

Most studies have evaluated the effect of plant extracts against CaOx due to their kidney stone type dominance identified in Moroccan epidemiological studies [26 - 29]. Atmani *et al.* tested the effect of the whole plant aqueous extract of *Herniaria hirsuta* on CaOx crystallization in human urine. From this research, the authors reported an increase in the number of crystals while their size decreased. Furthermore, this extract favored the formation of CaOx dehydrate rather than monohydrate crystals [29]. Oussama *et al.* investigated the *in vitro* effect of *Citrus limon* juice on CaOx crystallization in synthetic urine and proved a significant reduction in the rate of CaOx [30]. Using the same experimental approach (turbidimetric assay), Djareud *et al.* confirmed a slight inhibition of CaOx monohydrate crystallization (6%) using aqueous seed extract of *Hordeum vulgare*

[31]. In a recent study, Khouchlaa *et al.* tested *in vitro* the litholytic effect of *Zizyphus lotus* on CaOx and urate urinary calculi. They proved that fruit aqueous extract dissolved urate and CaOx. Whereas, the dissolution effect was more important on urate urinary calculi than CaOx [13].

Other plant extracts have been tested *in vitro* against cystine urinary calculi. The effect of aqueous extract of *Herniaria hirsute, Ammi visnaga, Opuntia ficus-indica, and Zea mays* separately showed a total dissolution of this calculi [10].

In Vivo Methods

In several *in vivo* researches, the authors used ethylene glycol (EG) to induce CaOx nephrolithiasis in rats (Table **1**). In this context, numerous plant extracts have been used to evaluate their effect against CaOx induced by EG such as *Crocus sativus, Zingiber officinale, Cynodon dactylon, Saccharum spontaneum, Herniaria hirsuta, Citrus limon,* and *Petroselinum sativum* . The results showed variability between plant extracts. Amin *et al.* tested the effect of stigmates aqueous extracts of *C. sativus* for its prophylactic and curative treatment. They proved that aqueous extract of this plant reduced malondialdehyde (MDA) levels and protected against ethylene glycol-induced CaOx nephrolithiasis [32]. In the same year, Lakshmi *et al.* investigated the antiurolithiasis effect of rhizomes ethanolic extracts of *Z. officinale* on EG-induced nephrolithiasis. From this research, it has been noted that this extract increased significantly urine output and reduced the levels ofcalcium, phosphate, uric acid, magnesium, and urea compared to control [33]. Furthermore, the ethanolic extract of *Z. Officinale* decreased crystals deposition in kidneys of calculogenic rats in curative and preventive treatment which has been also observed in rats treated with root hydroalcoholic extract of *C. dactylon* [33, 34]. Sathya and Kokilavani evaluated the anti-lithiasis effect of root ethanolic extract of *S. spontaneum* and reported a reduction in the level of xanthine oxidase, β-D-glucuronidasein, and n-acetyl --glucosaminidase [35]. Atmani *et al.* tried to mimic the use of *H. hirsuta* by the Moroccan population in *in vivo* experimental approach (nephrolitiasis rats induced by EG). They reported high magnesium levels, a smaller excretion of crystal stones, and no deposits of CaOx crystals in the kidneys of rats treated with the aqueous extract of the whole plant of *H. hirsuta* [36, 37]. Two studies evaluated the effect of *P. sativum* aqueous extract and reported a restoration of the urine pH to normal and a significant increase in the urine volume, magnesium, lipid peroxidation, and a decrease in crystals' CaOx content in kidneys [38, 39].

In other studies, the induction of CaOx in rats has been done by the use of glycolic acid added to their diet. In this case, the antiurolithiasis effect of aqueous seed extract of *A. visnage* on 3% glycolic acid-induced hyperoxaluria in rats has been evaluated by Khan and co-worker. The result showed that this extract decreased the urinary supersaturation in salts, a promoter of oxalocalcic lithiasis [40].

A vast majority of lithiasis is due to urinary metabolic abnormality induced by inadequate nutritional behavior and a defect of dieresis [41]. Jungers and collaborators reported this inadequate nutrition as consumption of refined sugar multiplied by 20, fat by 10, animal protein by 5, and salt by 3. At the same time, fiber consumption gets decreased [42]. Using these observations, researchers modified the rats' diets to induce nephrolithiasis.. Al Ali *et al.* modified rats' diet by givingtap water for 25 days of life processing with a high protein, carbohydrate, and caloric value (3400 cal/kg) diet and evaluated the effect of the aqueous hair extract of *Z. mays* in these rats. They reported that the aqueous extract of *Z. mays* did not influence citraturia, calciuria, or urinary pH values. However, combined with *Tribulus terrestris,* an increase in sodium, potassium, and urinary chlorine levels has been reported [43]. Thus, studying the synergistic effect of different plants which ensures the amelioration of antilithiasis effect is a very important pathway to treat kidney stones, and researches should be conducted to study the synergistic effect.

ANTILITHIATIC MECHANISM OF PHYTOMOLECULES

Despite the fact that there are numerous studies that have confirmed the pharmacological effects of Moroccan medicinal plant extracts against urolithiasis, a few of them have determined the mechanism behind the antilithiasic activity and the bioactive compounds responsible for this action. The complexity comes from the chemical composition of plant extracts used, which presents a diversity of molecules that can each act on different targets and at different stages of stone pathophysiology (Fig. **1**).

Changing Urine Parameters

Urinary pH is an important parameter for crystal stone formation and influences the chemical composition of kidney stones. It is known that uric acid stones tend to form in a low urinary pH (<5.05) and CaOx is independent in urinary pH [56, 57]. Plant extracts may act by altering urinary pH. This was reported with *C. limon,* which increased urinary pH from 6.7 to 6.9 [30]. Citrate has been mentioned by Penniston and co-workers as the main compound in the juice of *C. Limon*. This compound, freely filtered in the proximal tubule of the kidney, raised urinary pH which stopped the process of crystallization depending on urine pH [58, 59]. From these data, it can be concluded that *C. limon* can be used to inhibit the precipitation of uric acid stones and also to protect the formation of urolithiasis in hereditary stones by measuring morning urinary pH.

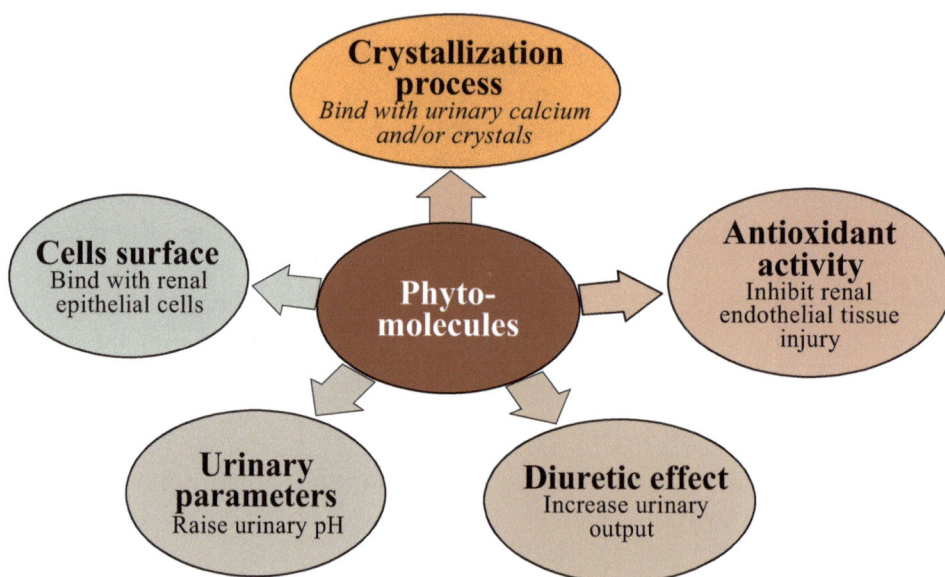

Fig. (1). Mechanism of action used by phytomolecules to prevent and/or treat kidney stones.

Diuretic

Urinary volume excreted plays an important role in the formation of urolithiasis. Low urine volumes are known to promote stone formation [35]. However, the increase in urine output decreases the saturation of crystals and prevent their precipitation at physiological pH [60]. Several authors have reported that *P.* and *Z. Officinale* increased significantly the urine output [32, 33] and this activity has been attributed to different compounds *viz.* cyaniding, quercetin [61, 62], luteolin [63], and pinene [64]. These compounds act by inhibing the Na^+/K^+ pump in renal epithelial cells, which increases diuresis [38].

Influence on The Crystallization Process

Plant extracts contain several active substances which have been described as inhibitors in different crystallization processes. Supersaturation is the leading process of crystallization [65]. Citrate reduced the supersaturation of urine by binding with urinary calcium. This effect reduced the free calcium concentration and inhibited the CaOx nucleation process [58]. The study of Vanachayangkul *et al.* proved that visnagin and khellin, the main compounds of *Ammi visnaga*, reduced significantly the deposition of CaOx crystals by blocking calcium activity [45]. Saponins showed an interesting antilithiasis effect as an inhibitor of uric acid by performing CaOx crystallization and their surfactant properties [19 - 66].

Cell Surface Adhesion

Crystal stones have been reported to possess a strong affinity for the membrane's renal epithelial cells and make a strong adhesion with these cells [60]. Phytomolecules involve different mechanisms to block this adhesion. Atmani *et al.* confirmed that bioactive compounds can block CaOx crystals' adhesion to the cell surface by blocking the attachment sites located in the cell surface or in the surface of the crystals [37]. The stability of this last complex (complexes of active compounds-crystals) could be ensured by hydrogen bonds and hydrophilic bonds between the functional groups of the active ingredients and carboxylic functions or amines. The complexes formed are much more soluble than the crystals themselves [10]. This action was also attributed to citric acid which exhibited both thermodynamic and kinetic mechanisms. Citrate inhibited crystal growth and aggregation by binding to the CaOx crystal surface and blocking its adhesion to renal epithelial cells [58]. In a recent study, Lai *et al.* reported that allicin, the main compound in *Allium sativum*, inhibited significantly the adhesion between CaOx adhesion crystals and renal cells [67].

Antioxidant Effect

Numerous studies have confirmed the ability of crystals to induce the production of reactive oxygen species (ROS) in kidney tissues [68, 69]. ROS production led to renal epithelial injury and increased the areas available for crystal attachment, eventual adhesion, and stone formation [70]. Natural polyphenols play an important role in the prevention of urolithiasis by inhibiting renal endothelial tissue injury. Quercetin, luteolin, and catechin have been reported to scavenge peroxide free radicals and inhibit lipid peroxidation by increasing the activity of endogenous antioxidants such as CAT, SOD, and GSH [60]. Bouzenna *et al.* reported the antioxidant activity of pinene. This compoud increased the level of GSH and decreased the levels of MDA [71].

CONCLUSION

This review reports the effect of medicinal plant extracts and their bioactive compounds as antilithogenic agents. Phytomolecules can act on different targets such as luteolin and pinene. These involve different mechanisms, including scavenging peroxide free radicals and increasing significantly the urine output.

Citrate has a dual action as it raises urinary pH and inhibits crystals' growth and aggregation process. Allicin inhibited the adhesion between crystals and renal cells. Visnagin and khellin reduced crystals deposition by blocking calcium activity. However, the synergistic effect of these bioactive compoundsshould be studied to ensure the amelioration of the antilithiasic effect. This is a very important pathway and current researches should investigate it in the study of synergistic effects with conventional chemotherapy. The *in vitro* and *in vivo* experiments reported in this review are limited. The plant extracts reported in this review have been used against two types of kidney stones: calcium oxalate and urate crystals. So, further investigation should be carried out on the effect of medicinal plant extracts and their bioactive compounds for the purpose to prevent and treat other types of crystal stones such as brushite. Studying the antilithiasic properties of plant extracts and their bioactive compounds also needs to include an increased number of toxicological assessments to guarantee the safety, efficacy, and quality of the prepared drugs.

CONSENT FOR PUBLICATION

Not Applicable.

CONFLICT OF INTEREST

The author declares no conflict of interest, financial or otherwise.

ACKNOWLEDGEMENTS

Declared none.

REFERENCES

[1]   Hmamouchi M. Moroccan medicinal and aromatic plants: Use, biology, ecology, chemistry, pharmacology, toxicity, lexicon. 1st ed. UK: Printing house Fédala 1999; p. 389.

[2]   Bellakhdar J. La pharmacopée marocaine traditionnelle Médecine ancienne et savoirs populaires. 1st ed. Lake Worth, FL: Ibis Press 1997; p. 764.

[3]   Iserin P, Chevallier A. Encyclopedia of medicinal plants. 2nd ed. New York: DK Publishing 1996; p. 335.

[4]   Wink M. Modes of action of herbal medicines and plant secondary metabolites. Medicines (Basel) 2015; 2(3): 251-86.
        [http://dx.doi.org/10.3390/medicines2030251] [PMID: 28930211]

[5]   Bruneton J. Pharmacognosy, Phytochemistry, Medicinal Plants. Lavoisier Technique & Documentation. Paris (In French). Paris; Secaucus, N.J.: Lavoisier Pub 1999; p. 1119.

[6]   Patel DK, Prasad SK, Kumar R, Hemalatha S. An overview on antidiabetic medicinal plants having insulin mimetic property. Asian Pac J Trop Biomed 2012; 2(4): 320-30.
        [http://dx.doi.org/10.1016/S2221-1691(12)60032-X] [PMID: 23569923]

[7]   Belayachi L, Aceves-Luquero C, Merghoub N, *et al.* Retama monosperma n-hexane extract induces cell cycle arrest and extrinsic pathway-dependent apoptosis in Jurkat cells. BMC Complement Altern

Med 2014; 14: 38-50.
[http://dx.doi.org/10.1186/1472-6882-14-38] [PMID: 24460687]

[8]   Khay EO, Bouyahya A, El Issaoui K, *et al.* Study of synergy between mentha pulegium essential oil, honey and bacteriocin-like inhibitory substance E204 against *Listeria monocytogenes* CECT4032 and *Escherichia coli* K12. IJCRBP 2016; 3(11): 29-35.
[http://dx.doi.org/10.20546/ijcrbp.2016.311.005]

[9]   Bouyahya A, Bakri Y, Khay EO, *et al.* Antibacterial, antioxidant and antitumor properties of Moroccan medicinal plants: A review. Asian Pacif Trop Dis 2017; 7: 57-64.
[http://dx.doi.org/10.12980/apjtd.7.2017D6-294]

[10]   Meiouet F, El Kabbaj S, Daudon M. Étude *in vitro* de l'activité litholytique de quatre plantes médicinales vis-à-vis des calculs urinaires de cystine. Prog Urol 2011; 21(1): 40-7.
[http://dx.doi.org/10.1016/j.purol.2010.05.009] [PMID: 21193144]

[11]   Jyothi MJ, Prathyusha S, Mohanalakshmi S, *et al.* Potent herbal wealth with litholytic activity: a review. IJIDD 2012; 2(2): 66-75.

[12]   Nagal A, Singla KR. Herbal resources with antiurolithiatic effects: a review. Indo Global J Pharm Sci 2013; 3(1): 6-14.

[13]   Khouchlaa A, Talbaoui A, El Yahyaoui El Idrissi A, *et al.* Détermination des composes phénoliques et évaluation de l'' activité litholitique *in vitro* sur la lithiase urinaire d'extrait de *Zizyphus lotus* L. d'origine marocaine. Phytotherapie (In press).
[http://dx.doi.org/10.1007/s10298-017-1106-3]

[14]   Geetha TS, Geetha N. Phytochemical screening, quantitative analysis of primary and secondary metabolites of cymbopogan citratus (DC) stapf leaves from Kodaikanal hills, Tamilnadu. Int J Pharm Tech Res 2014; 6(2): 521-9.

[15]   Ghourri M, Zidane L, Douira A. Catalogue des plantes médicinales utilisées dans le traitement de la lithiase rénale dans la province de Tan-Tan (Maroc saharien). Int J Biol Chem Sci 2013; 7: 1688-700.
[http://dx.doi.org/10.4314/ijbcs.v7i4.24]

[16]   Mikou K, Rachiq S, Jarrar Oulidi A. Ethnobotanical survey of medicinal and aromatic plants used by the people of Fez in Morocco. Phytotherapie 2016; 14(1): 35-43.
[http://dx.doi.org/10.1007/s10298-015-1013-4]

[17]   Salhi S, Fadli M, Zidane L, *et al.* Etude floristique et éthnobotanique des plantes médicinales de la ville de Kénitra (Maroc). Lazaroa 2010; 31: 133-46.
[http://dx.doi.org/10.5209/rev_LAZA.2010.v31.9]

[18]   Khouchlaa A, Tijane M, Chebat A, *et al.* Equête éthnopharmacologique des plantes des plantes utilisées dans le traitement de la lithiase urinaire au Maroc. Phytotherapie 2016; 15: 274-87.
[http://dx.doi.org/10.1007/s10298-016-1073-4]

[19]   Bouayyadi L, El Hafian M, Zidane L. Étude floristique et ethnobotanique de la flore médicinale dans la région du Gharb, Maroc. J Appl Biosci 2015; 93: 8760-9.
[http://dx.doi.org/10.4314/jab.v93i1.10]

[20]   El Hafian M, Benlamdini N, Elyacoubi H, *et al.* Étude floristique et ethnobotanique des plantes médicinales utilisées au niveau de la préfecture d'Agadir-Ida-Outanane (Maroc). J Appl Biosci 2014; 81: 7198-213.
[http://dx.doi.org/10.4314/jab.v81i1.8]

[21]   Lahsissene H, Kahouadji A, Tijane M, *et al.* Catalogue des plantes médicinales utilisées dans la region de Zaër (Maroc occidental). Lejeunia 2009; p. 186.

[22]   Hseini S, Kahouadji A. Etude ethnobotanique de la flore médicinale dans la region de Rabat (Maroc accidental). Lazaroa 2007; 28: 79-93.

[23]   Benlamdini N, Elhafian M, Rochdi A, *et al.* Étude floristique et éthnobotanique de la flore médicinale

du Haut Atlas oriental (Haute Moulouya). J Appl Biosci 2014; 78: 6771-87.
[http://dx.doi.org/10.4314/jab.v78i1.17]

[24]   Tahri NEL, Bastia A, Zidane L, *et al.* Etude ethnobotanique des plantes médicinales dans la province de Settat (Maroc). J For 2012; 12(2): 192-208.

[25]   Hachi M, Hachi T, Belahbib N, *et al.* Contribution à l'étude floristique et éthnobotanique de la flore médicinale utilisée au niveau de la ville de Khenifra (Maroc). International Journal of Innovation and Applied Studies 2015; 11: 754-70.

[26]   Dami F, Chouhani B, Elhabbani R, *et al.* Profil épidemiologique des patients lithiasiques. Nephrol Ther 2015; 11(5): 406.
[http://dx.doi.org/10.1016/j.nephro.2015.07.418]

[27]   Bouatia M, Benramdane L, Oulad Bouyahya Idrissi M, *et al.* An epidemiological study on the composition of urinary stones in Morocco in relation to age and sex. Afr J Urol 2015; 21: 194-7.
[http://dx.doi.org/10.1016/j.afju.2015.02.006]

[28]   Boumzaoued H, Laziri F, El Lekhlifi Z, *et al.* Prevalence of urinary lithiasis in the Moulay Ismail Military Hospital (Meknes-Morocco). J Mater Environ Sci 2015; 6(6): 1578-83.

[29]   Atmani F, Khan SR. Effects of an extract from *Herniaria hirsuta* on calcium oxalate crystallization *in vitro*. BJU International 2000 2000; 85(6): 621-5.

[30]   Oussama A, Touhami M, Mbarki M. *In vitro* and *in vivo* study of effect of lemon juice on urinary lithogenesis. Arch Esp Urol 2005; 58(10): 1087-92.
[http://dx.doi.org/10.4321/S0004-06142005001000019] [PMID: 16482864]

[31]   Djaroud S, Harrache D. Etude de l'effet de *Hordeum vulgare* sur la cristallisation de l'oxalate de calcium dans l'urine. Phytotherapie 2013; 11: 289-93.
[http://dx.doi.org/10.1007/s10298-013-0805-7]

[32]   Amin B, Feriz HM, Hariri AT, Meybodi NT, Hosseinzadeh H. Protective effects of the aqueous extract of Crocus sativus against ethylene glycol induced nephrolithiasis in rats. EXCLI J 2015; 14: 411-22.
[PMID: 26535035]

[33]   Lakshmi BVS, Divya V. Antiurolithiatic and antioxidant activity Of Zingiber Officinale rhizomes on ethylene glycol-induced urolithiasis in rats. Int J Adv Pharm Med Bioallied Sci 2015; 2(3): 148-53.

[34]   Khajavi Rad A, Hajzadeh MAR, Rajaei Z, Sadeghian MH, Hashemi N, Keshavarzi Z. Preventive effect of *Cynodon dactylon* against ethylene glycol-induced nephrolithiasis in male rats. Avicenna J Phytomed 2011; 1(1): 14-23.

[35]   Sathya M. Kokilavani. R. Antilithiatic activity of Saccharum spontaneum linn. on ethylene glycol induced lithiasis in rats. Int J Pharm Sci Res 2012; 3(9): 467-72.

[36]   Atmani F, Slimani Y, Mimouni M, Hacht B. Prophylaxis of calcium oxalate stones by *Herniaria hirsuta* on experimentally induced nephrolithiasis in rats. BJU Int 2003; 92(1): 137-40.
[http://dx.doi.org/10.1046/j.1464-410X.2003.04289.x] [PMID: 12823398]

[37]   Atmani F, Slimani Y, Mimouni M, Aziz M, Hacht B, Ziyyat A. Effect of aqueous extract from *Herniaria hirsuta* L. on experimentally nephrolithiasic rats. J Ethnopharmacol 2004; 95(1): 87-93.
[http://dx.doi.org/10.1016/j.jep.2004.06.028] [PMID: 15374612]

[38]   Moram GSE. Evaluation of anti-urolithiatic effect of aqueous extract of parsley (*Petroselinum sativum*) using ethylene glycol-induced renal calculi. World J Pharm Res 2016; 5(2): 1721-35.

[39]   Jafar S, Mehri L, Hadi B, *et al.* The antiurolithiasic and hepatocurative activities of aqueous extracts of *Petroselinum sativum* on ethylene glycol-induced kidney calculi in rats. Sci Res Essays 2012; 7: 1577-83.

[40]   Khan ZA, Assiri AM, Al-Afghani HM, Maghrabi TM. Inhibition of oxalate nephrolithiasis with *Ammi visnaga* (AI-Khillah). Int Urol Nephrol 2001; 33(4): 605-8.

[http://dx.doi.org/10.1023/A:1020526517097] [PMID: 12452606]

[41]   Daudon M, Traxer O, Lechevallier E, Saussine C. La lithogenèse. Prog Urol 2008; 18(12): 815-27.
       [http://dx.doi.org/10.1016/j.purol.2008.09.032] [PMID: 19033036]

[42]   Jungers P, Joly D, Blanchard A, Courbebaisse M, Knebelmann B, Daudon M. Lithiases rénales
       héréditaires monogéniques : récents acquis diagnostiques et thérapeutiques. Nephrol Ther 2008; 4(4):
       231-55.
       [http://dx.doi.org/10.1016/j.nephro.2007.12.005] [PMID: 18499551]

[43]   Al-Ali M, Wahbi S, Twaij H, Al-Badr A. *Tribulus terrestris*: preliminary study of its diuretic and
       contractile effects and comparison with Zea mays. J Ethnopharmacol 2003; 85(2-3): 257-60.
       [http://dx.doi.org/10.1016/S0378-8741(03)00014-X] [PMID: 12639749]

[44]   Sai Sindu P, Aparna M, Sravani B, *et al.* Evaluation of selected medicinal plants for antiurolithiatic
       activity. IJPSR 2012; 3(12): 5029-32.

[45]   Vanachayangkul P, Byer K, Khan S, Butterweck V. An aqueous extract of *Ammi visnaga* fruits and its
       constituents khellin and visnagin prevent cell damage caused by oxalate in renal epithelial cells.
       Phytomedicine 2010; 17(8-9): 653-8.
       [http://dx.doi.org/10.1016/j.phymed.2009.10.011] [PMID: 20036111]

[46]   Bhagavathula AS, Mahmoud Al-Khatib AJ, Elnour AA, Al Kalbani NM, Shehab A. *Ammi Visnaga* in
       treatment of urolithiasis and hypertriglyceridemia. Pharmacognosy Res 2014; 7(4): 397-400.
       [PMID: 26692756]

[47]   Beghalia M, Ghalem S, Allali H, *et al.* Inhibition of calcium oxalate monohydrate crystal growth using
       Algerian medicinal plants. J Med P Res 2008; 2: 66-70.

[48]   Sridharan B, Michael ST, Arya R, Mohana Roopan S, Ganesh RN, Viswanathan P. Beneficial effect of
       Citrus limon peel aqueous methanol extract on experimentally induced urolithic rats. Pharm Biol 2016;
       54(5): 759-69.
       [http://dx.doi.org/10.3109/13880209.2015.1079724] [PMID: 26452728]

[49]   Khajavi Rad A, Hadjzadeh MA, Rajaei Z, Mohammadian N, Valiollahi S, Sonei M. The beneficial
       effect of cynodon dactylon fractions on ethylene glycol-induced kidney calculi in rats. Urol J 2011;
       8(3): 179-84.
       [PMID: 21910095]

[50]   Sekkoum K, Cheriti A, Taleb S, *et al.* Inhibition Effect of Some Algerian Sahara Medicinal Plants on
       Calcium Oxalate Crystallization. Asian J Chem 2010; 22(4): 2891-7.

[51]   Atmani F, Khan SR. Effects of an extract from *Herniaria hirsuta* on calcium oxalate crystallization *in
       vitro*. BJU Int 2000; 85(6): 621-5.
       [http://dx.doi.org/10.1046/j.1464-410x.2000.00485.x] [PMID: 10759652]

[52]   Patel R, Shah JG. Effect of ethanolic extract of *Hordeum vulgare* seed on calcium oxalate deposition
       by surgericaly induced urolithiasis. J Pharm Sci Bioscientific Res 2017; 7(5): 335-40.

[53]   Mazdak H, Masoud Nikkar H, Ghanea L. Evaluation of *Raphanus sativus* effect on urinary pH. JRMS
       2007; 12: 58-61.

[54]   Ushakiran Ch. Evaluation and antiurolithiatic activity of *Raphanus sativus* extract by *in-vivo* on
       experimentaly induced urolithiasis in rats. Int J Pharm Pharm Ana 2017; 1(2): 71-8.

[55]   Baddade L, Elbir M, Mbarki M, *et al. Zizyphus lotus* Anti-lithiasis activity *in vitro* of aqueous extracts
       of pulp fruit in human urine. JMES 2019; 6: 520-5.

[56]   Kasote DM, Jagtap SD, Thapa D, Khyade MS, Russell WR. Herbal remedies for urinary stones used
       in India and China: A review. J Ethnopharmacol 2017; 203: 55-68.
       [http://dx.doi.org/10.1016/j.jep.2017.03.038] [PMID: 28344029]

[57]   Alelign T, Petros B. Kidney Stone Disease: An Update on Current Concepts. Adv Uro 2018; p.
       3068365.

[58]   Penniston KL, Nakada SY, Holmes RP, Assimos DG. Quantitative assessment of citric acid in lemon juice, lime juice, and commercially-available fruit juice products. J Endourol 2008; 22(3): 567-70.
[http://dx.doi.org/10.1089/end.2007.0304] [PMID: 18290732]

[59]   Rahman F, Birowo P, Widyahening IS, Rasyid N. Effect of citrus-based products on urine profile: A systematic review and meta-analysis. F1000 Res 2017; 6(6): 220.
[http://dx.doi.org/10.12688/f1000research.10976.1] [PMID: 28529700]

[60]   Ahmed S, Hasan MM, Khan H, Mahmood ZA, Patel S. The mechanistic insight of polyphenols in calcium oxalate urolithiasis mitigation. Biomed Pharmacother 2018; 106: 1292-9.
[http://dx.doi.org/10.1016/j.biopha.2018.07.080] [PMID: 30119199]

[61]   Jiménez-Ferrer E, Alarcón-Alonso J, Aguilar-Rojas A, *et al.* Diuretic effect of compounds from Hibiscus sabdariffa by modulation of the aldosterone activity. Planta Med 2012; 78(18): 1893-8.
[http://dx.doi.org/10.1055/s-0032-1327864] [PMID: 23150077]

[62]   Dinnimath BM, Jalalpure SS, Patil UK. Antiurolithiatic activity of natural constituents isolated from Aerva lanata. J Ayurveda Integr Med 2017; 8(4): 226-32.
[http://dx.doi.org/10.1016/j.jaim.2016.11.006] [PMID: 29169771]

[63]   Boeing T, da Silva LM, Mariott M, Andrade SF, de Souza P. Diuretic and natriuretic effect of luteolin in normotensive and hypertensive rats: Role of muscarinic acetylcholine receptors. Pharmacol Rep 2017; 69(6): 1121-4.
[http://dx.doi.org/10.1016/j.pharep.2017.05.010] [PMID: 29128789]

[64]   Bach T. Preclinical and clinical overview of terpenes in the treatment of urolithiasis. Eur Urol Suppl 2010; 9(12): 814-8.
[http://dx.doi.org/10.1016/j.eursup.2010.11.009]

[65]   Gupta S, Kanwar SS. Phyto-molecules for kidney stones treatment and management. Biochem Anal Biochem 2018; 7: 362.

[66]   Grases F, Costa-Bauzá A. Phytotherapy of renal lithiasis: myth and reality. Med Clin (Barc) 2000; 115(20): 779-82.
[http://dx.doi.org/10.1016/S0025-7753(00)71690-3] [PMID: 11171452]

[67]   Lai Y, Liang X, Zhong F, *et al.* Allicin attenuates calcium oxalate crystal deposition in the rat kidney by regulating gap junction function. J Cell Physiol 2019; 234(6): 9640-51.
[http://dx.doi.org/10.1002/jcp.27651] [PMID: 30378099]

[68]   Khan SR. Reactive oxygen species as the molecular modulators of calcium oxalate kidney stone formation: evidence from clinical and experimental investigations. J Urol 2013; 189(3): 803-11.
[http://dx.doi.org/10.1016/j.juro.2012.05.078] [PMID: 23022011]

[69]   Khan SR. Reactive oxygen species, inflammation and calcium oxalate nephrolithiasis. Transl Androl Urol 2014; 3(3): 256-76.
[PMID: 25383321]

[70]   Li X, Liang Q, Sun Y, *et al.* Potential mechanisms responsible for the antinephrolithic effects of an aqueous extract of *Fructus aurantii*. Evid Based Complement Alternat Med 2015.
[http://dx.doi.org/10.1155/2015/491409]

[71]   Bouzenna H, Hfaiedh N, Giroux-Metges MA, Elfeki A, Talarmin H. Potential protective effects of alpha-pinene against cytotoxicity caused by aspirin in the IEC-6 cells. Biomed Pharmacother 2017; 93: 961-8.
[http://dx.doi.org/10.1016/j.biopha.2017.06.031] [PMID: 28724214]

CHAPTER 8

Ethnobotanic, Phytochemical, and Biological Activities of *Aristolochia longa* L.: A Review

Amina El Yahyaoui El Idrissi, Aya Khouchlaa[*]**, Abdelhakim Bouyahya, Mereym El Fessikh, Youssef Bakri** and **M'hamed Tijane**

Department of Biology, Faculty of Science, Genomic Center of Human Pathologies, Faculty of Medicine, Laboratory of Human Pathologies Biology, Mohammed V University, Rabat, Morocco

Abstract: *Aristolochia longa* is a medicinal plant used in traditional Mediterranean pharmacopeia to treat different diseases. It shows significant anti-inflammatory, antidiabetic, antioxidant, antibacterial, and antitumoral pharmacological effects. The extracts of this plant are rich in bioactive molecules belonging to different chemical families such as limonene, aristolochic acid, β-caryophyllene, and deenax. However, excessive use of this plant causes severe toxicity to the user. The aim of the present review is to give particular emphasis on the most recent findings on biological effects of the major groups of *Aristolochia longa* components, their therapeutic use, and the active ingredient responsible for the toxicity of this plant, which constitutes a public health problem observed with it's wide use in cancer patients.

Keywords: *Aristolochia longa*, Anticancer, Antibacterial, Anti-inflammatory, Phytochemical, Toxicity.

INTRODUCTION

Aristolochiaceae is a family for *Aristolochia,* which includes nearly 500 species for most tropical, subtropical, and Mediterranean countries [1]. This family has been reported in the forests of America, Asia, Africa, Europe, and rarely in other countries with different species depending on the country *viz. Aristolochia indica* in India, *Aristolochia didyma* in South Americ, Aristolochia *clematitis* in Europe, *Aristolochia heppii* Merxm in East Africa, and is known in foreign languages as Isharmul (India), Wild dutchman's pip (Americ), Saracen (France), and chivide (East Africa) [2 - 4]. *Aristolochia longa* (*A. longa*), Mediterranean species in North Africa, known as Bereztem, was recommended since antiquity against ovarian insufficiency and snake bites [5].

[*] **Corresponding author Aya Khouchlaa:** Department of Biology, Faculty of Science, Genomic Center of Human Pathologies, Faculty of Medicine, Laboratory of Human Pathologies Biology, Mohammed V University, Rabat, Morocco; Tel: 00212674158222; E-mail: aya.khouchlaa@gmail.com

Anna Capasso (Ed.)

It was employed in traditional medicine to treat different diseases, such as cancer, diabetes, asthma, and skin and intestinal infections, using different parts of this plant with several forms as honey, milk, and jus [6 - 8]. Recently, it was increasing used against cancer and 44% of the Moroccan population studied approved healing by this plant [9].

Herbal remedies have a huge advantage over chemical treatment. Their secondary metabolites sowed several biological activities such as anti-tumor, antibacterial, antioxidant, antifungal, anti-inflammatory, and antidiabetic [1, 6 - 8, 10 - 14]. The biological properties of this plant have been attributed to a wide range of bioactive compounds, including polyphenols, flavonoids, alkaloids, tannic acid, and fatty acids [6]. In this way, studies showed that *A. longa* possessed actives molecules, such as aristolochic acid (AA), limonene, β-carotene, and palmitic acid (Fig. **1**), which have proven their pharmacological effects [10, 11, 15]. However, it is necessary to carefully determine the administered dose in order to be safe.

The aim of this review was, firstly, to make a synthesis of traditional therapeutical usages of *A. longa* in disease treatment and, secondly, to give data for the most recent findings on biological activity effect. Finally, we identified the major compounds from different parts of this plant and the mechanisms responsible for their action.

CLASSIFICATION AND BOTANICAL DESCRIPTION

1. Kingdom: Plantae
2. Branch: Angiosperms
3. Class: Magnoliopsida
4. Family: *Aristolochiaceae*
5. Genus: *Aristolochia*

A. longa is a perennial plant glabrescent (20-50cm of high), with slender stems, spreading, often ramose, with triangular, oval leaves, slightly heart-shaped (3-5cm of wide), corded base, margins whole and solitary green-brown flowers (Fig. **1**). It also gives very long fruits, compared to other species of aristolochia [16].

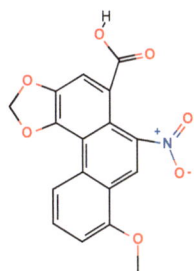

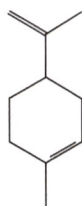

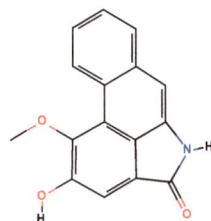

Aristolochic acid   Limonene   Aristolactam

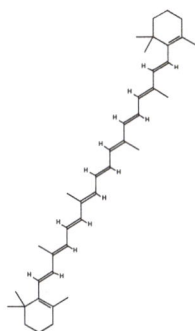

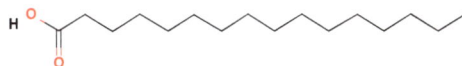

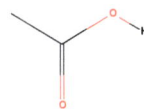

β-carotene   Palmitic acid   Acetic acid

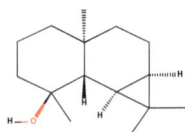

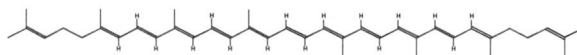

Maaliol   Lycopene

Fig. (1). Some phytochemicals identified in *A. longa*.

Ethnomedicobothany

A. longa has been used traditionally since antiquity and several ethnobotanical studies have published the use of this plant in illnesses treatment *viz*. cancer, diabetes, asthma, and digestive problems [9, 6, 17]. Table **1** summarizes the different parts and some traditional uses of *A. longa*. Depending on the area, the region, and the country, people use different parts of this plant and variable modes of preparation. The root has been used for asthma, palpitations of the aorta, antidote for snake bites, cancer treatment, and associated with Henne, used as a cataplasm, to treat skin diseases [18, 19]. Moreover, induced abortions in women are also treated with root *A. longa* [19]. The whole plant, in decoction, was used against intestinal affections and mixed with honey or salt butter in cases of cancer or with nigella, harmel, cumin, and pepper against stings and bites [19 - 21]. Other authors reported that this plant has been used in Morocco against "magic" [22]. However, the safe drug dose was not identified and this plant caused irreversible kidney damage along with hematuria, paralysis of limbs, and exposed people to the risk of carcinogenicity [23]. According to each country's action plan, it was established that *A. longa* was available for open sale in Morocco, controlled used in Algeria, prohibited in Australia, and restricted in Europe. Thus, the European Commission has prohibited *Aristolochia* species and use of their preparations in cosmetic products [7, 24, 25].

Table 1. Ethnobotanical data of traditional used of *A. longa*..

Countries	Used Part	Preparation Methods	Therapeutic Used	References
Morocco	nd	nd	Pathological digestive	[17]
	Root	Cataplasm, decoction	Skin diseases, asthma, palpitations of the aorta, constipation and intestinal infections, asthma, antidote for snake bites, emetico-cathartic and diuretic, induce abortion in women	[19]
	Whole plant	Cataplasm	Skin affections, intestinal affections	[20, 21]
	Rhizome	Powder , decoction	Diabetes	[23]
	Whole or in part	Decoction, Infusion, Powder, Maceration	Cancer, kidney diseases, diabetes, menstrual problems, appetite.	[9]
	Rhizome	Cataplasm	Cancer, diabetes, and asthma	[18]
Algeria	Root	Raw	Breast cancer	[26]
		nd	Astringent, anti-rheumatic	[27]
	Tuber	nd	Anti-inflammatory, antiseptic	[28]

Phytochemistry of *A. longa*

During the last years, there has been a growing interest in the effect of this plant following numerous toxicities declared by the poison control center [9]. The biological properties of *A. longa* have been attributed to a wide range of bioactive compounds, including polyphenols, flavonoids, alkaloids, tannic acid, essential oil compounds [29 - 31]. An overview of bioactive compounds for each part of *A. longa* was presented thereafter.

Major Compounds, Including Phenols, Flavonoids, Alkaloids, Saponins

In the medicinal plant, the partition of active compounds differed between different parts of the plant, the type of extract used, and the place and season of growing [7, 8]. The phytochemical composition of *A. longa* has not been widely discussed and few studies have explored the chemical composition of this plant. Table **2** summarizes the distribution of major compounds in the aerial part, *i.e.*, leaf, tuber, fruit, and roots of *A. longa*. These compounds are known for their biological activities, including radical scavenging properties due to their hydroxyl groups [27]. The content of phenolic compounds has been expressed in gallic acid equivalents (GAE). Total phenolics in root were the major compounds with 6.07 mg/g followed by the fruit part [6 - 11]. The content of flavonoids varied and the high amount was found in root extract (0.81 mg/g) [27]. Catechin tannins, C-heterosides, carbohydrates, and saponins were present in *A. longa* root extract with a qualitative test [6]. Thus, the quantities were not identified.

Studies were released to determine the chemical composition of the different parts of *A. longa* [7-10-28]. β-caryophyllene and caryophyllene were identified in the essential oil of *A. longa* from the aerial parts, which were involved in antibacterial and antioxidant activities [32 - 34]. Aneb *et al.* identified a high amount of limonen-6-ol and 9-, Octadecane in tuber that possessed, respectively, anti-inflammatory and antibacterial activities [10, 35, 36]. Furthermore, limonen-6-ol demonstrated antioxidant and anticancer properties and was commonly used in perfumes, household cleaners, and foods [37]. Fruit of *A. longa* consists of lycopene and β-carotene [11]. These are the most important antioxidants in the diet, and may lower the risk of certain diseases, such as cancer [38]. In the leaf, four compounds were identified, deenax, diisoctylftalate, acetic acid, and 3,3,5,5-tetramethyl-8-(3-methylbutyl)-6,7-dihydro-2H-s-indacen-1-one [28]. Acetic acid has been shown to be antifungal, antibacterial, antioxidant, antidiabetic, and antitumoral [39 - 41]. The other compounds were not isolated and tested to prove their biological effects. Thus, more research must be conducted to investigate these effects and exploit the unexploited part of this plant. AA, nitrophenanthrene carboxylic acid, was the main constituent reported in a wide range of *Aristolochiaceae* species, and varied in the amount among species. This alkaloid can be found in other genus belonging to the *Aristolochiaceae* family, like Asarum and Bragantia [42]. AA was identified in aqueous tuber extract and essential oil of *A. longa* and also presented in root [11, 15, 32]. 13 AAs of natural origin have been identified from different plants of family *Aristolochiaceae* species [44]. Researchers showed that *A. bracteolate* L. contains a high quantity of AA-II (49.03 g/kg) compared to *A. debilis* (0.18 g/kg), *A. fangchi* (0.22 g/kg), and *A. manshuriensi* (1.0 g/kg). The same remark was identified for AA-I with a high amount of 12.98 g/kg for *A. bracteolate* L. compared to the other species

[43]. These compounds (AA) possessed immunostimulatory, anti-inflammatory, and antibacterial properties [11]. It was worth noting that, for *A. longa*, neither the quantities nor the type of AA has been identified. Thus, more investigation must be done.

Table 2. Distribution of major bioactive compounds in various parts of *A. longa*.

Used Part	Major Component	Content	References
Aerial parts aqueous extract	Total phenolic	396*	[11]
	Flavonoids	9.92*	
	Flavones and flavonols	27.40*	
	Tannins	54.4*	
	β-carotene	0.393*	
	Lycopene	0.0213*	
Aerial parts essential oil	β-caryophyllene	-	[32]
	Caryophyllene	-	
Fruit aqueous extract	Total phenolic	518.54*	[11]
	Flavonoids	5.81*	
	Flavones and flavonols	21.64*	
	Tannins	14.14*	
	β-carotene	0.023*	
	Lycopene	0.015*	
Root phenolic extract	Total phenolic	1.47**	[27]
	Flavonoids	0.81**	
	Flavonols	0.41**	
Root aqueous extract	Total phenolic	6.07**	[6]
	Flavonoids	-	
	Catechin tannins	-	
	Carbohydrates	-	
	C-heterosides	-	
	Saponins	-	

(Table 2) cont.....

Used Part	Major Component	Content	References
Tuber aqueous extract	Total phenolic	293.82*	[11]
	Flavonoids	4.86*	
	Flavones and flavonols	23.16*	
	Tannins	21.2*	
	β-carotene	0.039*	
	Aristolochic acid	-	[28]
Tuber extract	(2'-Nitro-2'-propenyl) cyclohexane	19.16§	[10]
	Heptadecane, 2,6,10,15-tetramethyl-	5.58§	
	Cycloheptane, 4-methylene -1-methyl-2-(2-methyl-1-propen-1-yl)-1-vinyl	7.07§	
	Cholestan-3-ol, 2-methylene-, (3à,5à)-	17.32§	
	d-Glycero-d-ido-heptose	15.42§	
	-Octadecenal	8.36§	
	1-Gala-1-ido-octose	65.66§	
	Octadecane	34.33§	
	Limonen-6-ol, pivalate	55.84§	
	Permethylated	73.02§	
Tuber essential oil	Lycopene, 1,2-dihydro-1-hydroxy-	-	[15]
	Aristolochic acid	-	
	3,3,5,5-tetramethyl-8-(3-methylbutyl)-6,7-dihydro-2H-s-indacen-1-one	-	
Leaf essential oil	Aristolochic acid	-	
	Diethylhexylphthalate	-	
	3,3,5,5-tetramethyl-8-(3-methylbutyl)-6,7-dihydro-2H-s-indacen-1-one	-	
	Butylated hydroxytoluene	-	
	acetic acid	-	

*: μg/mg, **: mg/g, §: %, (-) unspecified quantities

Fatty Acid Composition

The other classes of phytochemicals determined in *A. longa* were fatty acids composition and few studies investigated their partition in this plant. Their partition, including saturated, monounsaturated, and polyunsaturated fatty acids, differed between different parts of this plant (Table **3**). Dhouioui *et al.* confirmed a high content of saturated fatty acids in roots. Palmitic acid was the fatty acid found the most in root hexane extracts and stems essential oil, accounting for 34.22% and 40.23%, respectively [28, 45]. This acid showed an anti-tumor and antimicrobial activity [46, 47]. Leaves methanolic extract was very rich in linoleic acid (62.45%) [28], which possessed medicinal properties such as anti-inflammatory, antiandrogenic, cancer preventive, insectifuge, and antibacterial activities [47, 48]. Cherif *et al.* proved that linolenic acid was the most abundant fatty acid in rizhome methanol extracts, which was responsible for anti-inflammatory activities and had a potent antibacterial activity [28, 49, 50]. Thus, *A. longa* also contains small quantities of essentials oil compounds, such as arachidic acid, caprylic acid, and lauric acid, which can be effective with the synergy between them and the high amounts of the main constituents. Recent researches demonstrated the distribution of other long fatty acids such as 9,12,15-Octadecatrienoic acid, methyl ester, (Z, Z, Z); 3-Hexadecyloxycarbonyl-5-(2-hydroxyethyl)-4-methylimidazolium ion and trans-Z-à-Bisabolene epoxide [10]. In further researches, these molecules must be isolated and tested for different biological effects since the extracts and essential oil showed anti-inflammatory, anti-tumor, antibacterial activities. Other authors showed that maaliol and eremophilone were found in a high amount in March. While other compounds, such as isospathulenol and 2,3-Dihydro-benzofuran, were not present during this period [45]. The season factor must be taken into consideration, which could affect metabolic pathways of phytochemicals composition in the same part of the plant. However, other researches must be conducted for the identification of fatty acids influenced by the season in other parts of this plant.

Table 3. Comparison of the fatty acid composition of *A. longa* (compositions are expressed in %).

Fatty Acid Type Extract	C10:0	C12:0	C16:0	C16:1 w-7	C17:0	C18:0	C18:1 w-9	C18:2 w-6	C18:3 w-3	C20:0	C22:0	Reference
Root hexane extract	0.6	0.26	34.22	2.85	1.12	12.06	24.26	19.58	0.10	1.81	2.37	[45 - 28]
Root essential oils	-	-	22.97	-	-	-	-	-	-	-	-	
Aerial parts hexane extract	2.22	3.85	15.59	6.04	-	16.35	7.01	-	25.31	-	-	[45]

(Table 3) cont.....

Fatty Acid Type Extract	C10:0	C12:0	C16:0	C16:1 w-7	C17:0	C18:0	C18:1 w-9	C18:2 w-6	C18:3 w-3	C20:0	C22:0	Reference
Leaves methanolic extract	-	-	18.02	-	-	-	-	62.45	12.32	2.52	-	[28]
Leaves essential oils	-	-	-	-	-	-	-	-	34.01	-	-	
Stems methanolic extract	-	-	22.28	-	-	-	-	33.33	34.40	-	-	
Stems essential oils	-	-	40.23	-	-	-	-	-	-	-	-	
Rhizomes methanolic extract	-	-	20.87	-	-	-	-	11.53	35.07	-	-	
Rhizomes essential oils	-	-	22.87	-	-	-	-	-	-	-	-	

(-) unspecified quantities

PHARMACOLOGICAL AND BIOLOGICAL ACTIVITIES OF *A. LONGA* COMPOUNDS

During the last decades, *A. longa* has attracted much attention and has been the subject of several pharmacological studies worldwide. Nevertheless, the therapeutic benefits of *A. longa* compounds and/or extracts have been highlighted by a few experimental models. Table **4** summarizes the biological properties of different parts of *A. longa* through *in vitro* and *in vivo* studies.

Anti-tumor Activities

On one hand, *in vitro* antitumoral studies of aqueous root extract of *A. longa* proved their effect against tumor cells. Benarba *et al.* demonstrated that aqueous root extract of *A. longa* induced apoptosis of Burkitt's lymphoma cells (BL41) with an IC_{50} estimated at 15,63 µg/mL [1]. Recently, root aqueous extract of this plant against two breast cancer cell lines, MDA-MB-231 and HBL100, showed IC50=97µg/mL and IC50=40µg/mL [14]. Legault *et al.* demonstrated that β-caryophyllene stimulates apoptosis and suppresses tumor growth [51].

Table 4. Overview of major bioactive effects of *A. longa* preparations in different experimental models.

Biological Activities	Used Part	Type of Extract	Used Test	Effects	References
Antitumoral	Root	Aqueous extract	*In vitro* test against Burkitt's lymphoma BL41 cells.	IC_{50} = 15,63 μg/mL	[1]
		Aqueous extract	*In vitro* test against Breast cancer cell lines MDA-MB-231 and HBL100.	IC_{50} = 97μg/mL against MDA cells IC_{50} = 40μg/mL against HBL cells	[14]
		Aqueous extract	*In vivo* test against breast cancer postmenopausal women	Increasing serum creatinine, urea, and uric.	[57]
		Aristolochic acid and Aristolactam Ia from benzene root extract	*In vitro* testing against the murine leukemia P-388 (9PS)	Active *in vitro* on P-388 lymphocytic leukemia system	[54]
	Tuber	Hexane	*In vitro* test against RD*, BSR* and Vero* cancerous cell lines	IC_{50} = 30μg/mL against RD IC_{50} = 18μg/mL against BSR Poor cytotoxicity against Vero	
		Dichloromethane		IC_{50} = 15μg/mL against RD IC_{50} = 60μg/mL against BSR Poor cytotoxicity against Vero	[10]
		Methanol		IC_{50} = 30μg/mL against RD IC_{50} = 350μg/mL against BSR Poor cytotoxicity against Vero	
	Rhizome	Aqueous extract	*In vivo* study in Wistar rats gingival tumorigenesis induced	Pro-inflammatory reactions in the oral cavity, lungs with a high number of eosinophil.	[13]
Antibacterial	Aerial parts	Hexane extract	Agar well diffusion method (*Rhodococcus equi, Rhodococcus sp* GK1, *Rhodococcus sp* GK3)	φ=26mm against R. equi φ=26mm against R. sp GK3	
		Dichloromethane		φ=30mm against R. equi φ=25mm against R. sp GK1	[10]
		Methanol		No significant activity observed	

(Table 4) cont.....

Biological Activities	Used Part	Type of Extract	Used Test	Effects	References
	Aerial parts (Ap), Fruits (F) and tubers (T)	Acetone	Agar diffusion method (*E. coli* ATCC 25922, *P. aeruginosa* ATCC 27853, S. *aureus* ATCC 25923, *B. cereus* ATCC 10876)	Unable to inhibit *E. coli* φ=17mm against *P. aeruginosa* (Ap) φ=11mm against *S. aureus* (Ap) φ=15mm against *B. cereus* (Ap) φ=11mm against *P. aeruginosa* (F) φ=11mm against *S. aureus* (F) φ=14.5mm against B. *cereus* (F) φ=7mm against *B. cereus* (T)	[11]
		Methanol		Unable to inhibit *E. coli* φ=15mm against *P. aeruginosa* (F) φ=17mm against *S. aureus* (F) φ=14mm against *B. cereus* (F) φ=9mm against *B. cereus* (T)	
		Water		Unable to inhibit *E. coli* φ=15mm against *S. aureus* (Ap) φ=8mm against *S. aureus* (F)	
		Acetone	Microdillution method against (P. *aeruginosa* ATCC 27853, *S. aureus* ATCC 25923, *B. cereus* ATCC 10876)	MIC=12.5mg/mL against all bacteria (Ap, F, T)	
		Methanol		MIC=3.12mg/mL against *P. aeruginosa, S. aureus* (F) MIC=6.25mg/mL against *B. cereus* (F)	
		Water		MIC=50mg/mL against *P. aeruginosa* (Ap) MIC=125mg/mL against *S. aureus* (Ap)	
	Root	Essential oil	Disc diffusion methods (*E. faecium* ATCC 19434, *S. agalactiae, S. aureus* ATCC 6538, *E. coli* ATCC 8739, *S. typhimurium* ATCC 14028)	φ=35.9mm against *E. faecium* φ=41.8mm against *S. agalactiae* φ=13.2mm against *S. aureus* φ=0mm against *E. coli* φ=9.4mm against *S. typhimurium*	[45]

(Table 4) cont.....

Biological Activities	Used Part	Type of Extract	Used Test	Effects	References
Antifungal	Aerial parts, fruits and tubers	Acetone, methanol, and water	*In vitro* fungi tested (*Aspergillus flavus* NRRL 391, *Aspergillus niger* 2CA 936, *Candida albicans* ATCC1024)	All extract were unable to inhibit the growth of the fungi tested	[11]
	Root	Essential oil	*In vitro* disc diffusion method against *Candida albicans* ATTCC10231	ϕ=12,1mm	[45]
Anti-inflammatory	Aerial parts, fruits and tubers	Acetone, methanol, and water	*Invitro* protein denaturation methods	Acetone aerial parts=78.35% Fruit methanolic extract=68.04%	[11]
Antidiabetic	Root	Ethyl acetate	*In vitro* α-Glucosidase and $\square$-Galactosidase inhibitory activities	IC50=1.11mg/mL against α-Glucosidase IC50>5mg/mL against α-Galactosidase	[8]
		Methanol		IC50=2.37mg/ml against α-Glucosidase IC50>5mg/ml against α-Galactosidase	
		Water		IC50>5mg/ml against α-Glucosidase IC50>5mg/ml against α-Galactosidase	
Antioxidant	Aerial part (Ap), fruit (F), tuber (T)	Acetone (A), methanol (M), and water (W)	DPPH radical scavenging activity	IC50=182.59μg /mL (ApA) IC50=547.29μg /mL (FA) IC50=311.27μg /mL (TA) IC50=55.04μg /mL (ApM) IC50=186.21μg /mL (FM) IC50=514.58μg /mL (TM) IC50=157.13μg /mL (ApW) IC50=145.15μg /mL (FW) IC50=198.06μg /mL (TW)	[11]

(Table 4) cont.....

Biological Activities	Used Part	Type of Extract	Used Test	Effects	References
			β-Carotene-linoleic acid assay	57% for ApA 36% for FA 23% for TA 33% for ApM 28% for FM 22% for TM 30% for ApW 16% for FW 12% for TW	
			FRAP* Assay	EC50=1.23µg /mL (ApA) EC50=2.42µg /mL (FA) EC50=2.49µg /mL (TA) EC50=0.20µg /mL (ApM) EC50=1.53µg /mL (FM) EC50=2.64µg /mL (TM) EC50=0.63µg /mL (ApW) EC50=1.86µg /mL (FW) EC50=5.99µg /mL (TW)	
	Root	Phenolic extract	DPPH radical scavenging activity	IC50=90.16µg /mL	[28]
		Ethyl acetate (Ea), methanol (M) and water (W)	DPPH radical scavenging activity	IC50=220.80µg /mL (Ea) IC50=199.35µg/mL (M) IC50=354.60µg/mL (W)	[8]
			ABTS Radical Scavenging Assay	IC50=103.62µg/mL (Ea) IC50=61.58µg/mL (M) IC50=144.40µg/mL (W)	
Immunos-timulatory	Rhizome	Aqueous extract	*In vivo* immunomodulatory activity	Increase in primary titer values of antibodies and high number of lymphocytes	[12]
Toxicity	Root	Aqueous extract	*In vivo* acute oral toxicity at dose limited 5g/kg in albino rats	No toxic effect	[1]
		Powder	*In vivo* protective effect of *A. longa* on acute hepatotoxicity induced by lead in albino rats at 10g/kg of diet	Decreasing oxidative stress and decreasing of alteration of the liver tissue	[71]
	Rhizome	Aqueous extract	*In vivo* acute oral toxicity in albino rats at doses of 1,25 and 2,25g/kg/day for 3 and 6 weeks	At 1,25g/kg: no toxic effect At 2,25g/kg: AST*: 45 U/L; ALT*: 80 U/L; Creatinine: 4mg/L	[12]

IC$_{50}$: Half maximal inhibitory concentration; EC$_{50}$: Half maximal effective concentration; ϕ: Zone of inhibition.

It was the same as lycopene and palmitic acid, which inhibited cell proliferation and induced apoptosis by activation mitochondrial Ca^{2+}-dependent pore, causing the release of cytochromes c by mitochondria [38, 52]. Other mechanisms of action can be attributed to compounds in aqueous extract of *A. longa* who activated the intrinsic pathway of apoptosis by the activation of caspase-3/7, PARP, caspase-9 cleavage and the release of reactive oxygen species by eosinophil [1, 13, 53]. Other authors studied the cytotoxic activities of *A. longa* tuber extract against 3 cancerous lines. Hexane and dichloromethane extract presented significant inhibiting effects with a significant cytotoxic activity, which agrees with previous researches in the family of *Aristolochiaseae* especially two active principals, AA and aristolactam [54, 55]. On the other hand, an *in vivo* study in Wistar rats gingival tumorigenesis exhibited pro-inflammatory reactions in the oral cavity and lungs with a high number of eosinophil's [13]. This effect can be attributed to the major compounds of *A. longa* who possess immunostimulatory propriety [56]. Other *in vivo* tests against breast cancer postmenopausal women showed that *A. longa* aqueous extract increased serum creatinine, urea, and uric and may be detrimental for kidney function in breast cancer patients [57]. However, the mechanism inducing the reduction of renal function was unknown. Altogether, these reports provided evidence that *A. longa* could be considered as a source of natural biomolecules to treat cancer. However, the safe dose must be known.

Antibacterial and Antifungal Activities

Antibacterial activities of *A. longa* have been studied against several bacterial strains. Dhouioui *et al.* tested the effect of essential oil of *A. longa* from root against *Enterococcus faecium, Streptococcus agalactiae, Staphylococcus aureus, Escherichia coli,* and *Salmonella typhimurium*. The highest activity was observed against *S. agalactiae,* which was particularly sensitive with an inhibition zone of 41.8mm [45]. The mechanism of action can be attributed to compounds in *A. longa* essential oil that induced leakage of intracellular sodium and alteration of membrane potential, which cause an increase in the membrane permeability and a loss in the respiratory and enzymatic activities [58]. Other studies confirmed that palmitoleic acid, oleic acid, linolenic acid, and arachidonic acid exhibited the inhibition of an essential component of bacterial fatty acid synthesis, enoyl-acyl carrier protein reductase [47]. However, gram-negative bacteria exhibited resistance against the essential oil *of A. longa* related to the restrictive outer membrane barrier [45]. *A. longa* extracts also revealed variable levels of antimicrobial activity against Gram-positive and Gram-negative bacterial strains. Hexane and dichlorometane extracts from aerial parts of *A. longa* have shown a strong growth inhibition effect on all *Rhodococcus* tested, which may be related to the high content in linoleic acid chloride; oleic acid, and limonene-6-ol in this plant while no significant activity was observed with methanolic extract [10]. Studies reported a high content of alkaloids, which have an antimicrobial capacity exercised through interference with the process of DNA replication and RNA transcription [59]. In addition, studies proved that polyphenols combined with the peptidoglycan and phospholipid bilayer of the outer membrane of bacteria, reduce the integrity of the cell membrane. These compounds affect the activities of bacterial intracellular enzymes by reacting with the amino and carboxyl groups of proteins as well as the chelating transition metal ion to inhibit the growth of the bacteria [41]. Indeed, the variation of these results was influenced by extract type, bacterial membrane structure, season, and concentration and chemical composition of extracts.

Other studies reported the effects of *A. longa* extracts on the growth of fungi species. They demonstrated that all extracts (Acetone, methanol, and water) were unable to inhibit the growth of the fungi tested (*Aspergillus flavus* NRRL 391, *Aspergillus niger* 2CA 936, *Candida albicans* ATCC1024) [11]. However, essential oil from root inhibited *C. albicans* ATTCC10231 (12,1mm) [45] due to the potent activity of an alkane, octadecane [60]. Furthermore, the mechanisms thought to be responsible for phenolic toxicity to microorganisms include enzyme inhibition by the oxidized compounds [61]. These results might be considered as a source of natural biomolecules against bactericides.

Antidiabetic Activities

Rare studies evaluated the antidiabetic activities of this plant. Recently, an *in vitro* model was investigated using β-Glucosidase and β-Galactosidase inhibitory activities effect of *A. longa* indicated that the fraction of ethyl acetate and methanol of roots present the most efficient activities against β-Glucosidase with IC50 values of 1.112 and 2.378mg/mL [8]. Other species in the same family, *A. indica*, showed an excellent antihyperglycemic activity which was correlated with high quantities of phenolic compounds known by their capacity to inhibit the activities of carbohydrate-hydrolyzing enzymes because of their ability to bind to proteins [62]. Moreover, flavonoids have been known to possess high inhibitory potential towards *β*-Glucosidase in both *in vitro* and *in vivo* studies [63]. Indeed, β-caryophyllene modulated the activities of key enzymes by increasing insulin secretion and restoring glucose homeostasis [64]. Furthermore, Chen *et al.* proved that acetic acid regulated the concentration of blood by delaying gastric emptying, inhibiting disaccharidase activity, improving insulin sensitivity, and finely promoting the production of glycogen [41].

Antioxidant Activities

Numerous studies investigated the ability of *A. longa* extract to scavenge free radical using 2,2-diphenyl-1-picrylhydrazyl (DPPH) scavenging activity and ABTS methods, β-Carotene-linoleic acid assay. On one hand, an *in vitro* research showed that aerial parts methanol extract and root phenolic extract exhibited the highest antioxidant capacity of DPPH with IC_{50} = 55,04 µg/mL and IC_{50} = 55,04 µg/mL, respectively [11 - 27]. Recently, an aqueous fraction of this herb exhibited the highest antioxidant activity for DPPH with IC_{50} = 125.4 µg/mL [8]. However, *A. indica* showed an important antioxidant activity (IC_{50}=7.32 µg/mL) due to the active molecule isolated, β-sitostero [62]. In ABTS methods, aqueous fraction showed the highest antioxidant activity with IC_{50} = 65.23 µg/mL, which is analog to *A. bracteolate* methanolic extract. The presence of phenolic compounds might be the reason for reducing power and also with the synergy effect with other compounds [8 - 65]. On the other hand, an *in vivo* study showed that this plant was beneficial to treat lead-induced oxidative stress in the heart due to the high amount of radical scavenging compounds in *A. longa* with the proton-donating ability [8 - 66].

Anti-inflammatory Activities

Only one *in vivo* study tested extracts of *A. longa* with protein denaturation methods. Acetone extracts from aerial parts have the highest inhibition of protein denaturation (78.35%), which probably involved alteration electrostatic hydrogen, hydrophobic, and disulfide bonding [11]. Rufino showed the anti-inflammatory effect of limonene, which increased extracellular signal-regulated Kinase and reduced p38 phosphorylation, and caused the activation of caspases inducing inhibiting inflammation [36]. Indeed, linoleic acid inhibited the transcription of pro-inflammatory cytokines by the upregulation of peroxisome proliferator receptor- α/γ [67]. AA had direct interaction with phospholipase A2, which leads to the formation of local inflammatory mediators *viz.* prostaglandins, leukotrienes, and thromboxanes [68].

Immunostimulatory Activities

Aqueous extract of *A. longa* showed a stimulatory effect of both humoral and cellular immune function. It was identified to have a high number of lymphocytes in different organs with a significant increase in haemagglutinating antibody titer and delayed-type hypersensitivity [12]. The mechanism of action was related to the sensibility of T-lymphocytes with terpenoids in *A. longa* induced conversion to lymphoblast. This secreted a variety of pro-inflammatory lymphokines, attracting more scavenger cells to the site of reaction [69, 70].

Toxicity Effect

In traditional folks, *A. longa* caused many side effects, including breathing problems, vomiting, and diarrhea. It has been considered nephrotoxic, carcinogenic, and mutagenic [43]. According to the results of the Benarba study, the aqueous extract of this plant was safe at 5g/kg [1]. However, these results were contradictory with the study of Benzakour, who showed significant toxicity on the liver, intestine, and kidney when administrated at 2,25g/kg/day [12]. These alterations may be due to the defective activation of antioxidative enzymes and mitochondrial damage caused by AA tubular toxicity impaired regeneration of proximal tubular epithelial cells and apoptosis, secondary to caspase-3 activation, may be involved [28, 56]. Other studies investigated the protective effect of *A. longa* on acute hepatotoxicity induced by lead (Pb) and showed that this plant inhibited hepatic damage caused by Pb. The mechanism of action may be related to the reduction of free radicals induced by Pb [71]. Furthermore, AA, injected into the patient for 0.1mg/kg/day, was too toxic to the kidney and has been limited in clinical applications because of its severe nephrotoxic activity [72]. Further *in vivo* experiments should be conducted for the highest compounds in *A. longa*, AA to determine a safe clinical dose. Indeed, the effect of this molecule may be less toxic with a synergistic effect of small quantities of compounds in extract of *A. longa* than this compound that can accomplish them individually.

CONCLUSION

Bioactive compounds, other than aristolochic acid, from *A. longa,* possess promising pharmacological activities. Maaliol, lycopene, limonene, and *β*-caryophyllene being identified in several essential oils, organic and aqueous extracts of this plant, provided evidence that *A. longa* with various biological effects could be considered as a source of natural biomolecules to have beneficial effects on human health. However, rare were researches that studied the synergy effect of these bioactive compounds with other components, including conventional drugs. This is a very important way and current researches should be conducted in the study of synergistic effects with conventional chemotherapy. In addition, further *in vivo* investigations are necessary to study the efficacy of compounds and to ensure the development of a safe potential drug to treat different diseases.

CONSENT FOR PUBLICATION

Not Applicable.

CONFLICT OF INTEREST

The author declares no conflict of interest, financial or otherwise.

ACKNOWLEDGEMENTS

Declared none.

REFERENCES

[1]   Benarba B, Ambroise G, Aoues A, *et al. Aristolochia longa* aqueous extract triggers the mitochondrial pathways of apoptosis in BL41 Burkitt's lymphoma cells. IJGP 2012; 6: 45-9.
        [http://dx.doi.org/10.4103/0973-8258.97128]

[2]   Heinrich M, Chan J, Wanke S, Neinhuis C, Simmonds MS. Local uses of *Aristolochia* species and content of nephrotoxic aristolochic acid 1 and 2--a global assessment based on bibliographic sources. J Ethnopharmacol 2009; 125(1): 108-44.
        [http://dx.doi.org/10.1016/j.jep.2009.05.028] [PMID: 19505558]

[3]   Dey A, Natha De J. *Aristolochia indica* L.: A Review. Asian J Plant Sci 2011; 10(2) (Suppl.): 108-16.
        [http://dx.doi.org/10.3923/ajps.2011.108.116]

[4]   Sewani-Rusike CR. Plants of Zimbabwe used as anti-fertility agents. Afr J Tradit Complement Altern Med 2010; 7(3) (Suppl.): 253-7.
        [http://dx.doi.org/10.4314/ajtcam.v7i3.54785] [PMID: 21461153]

[5]   Carvalho BM, Santos JD, Xavier BM, *et al.* Snake venom PLA2s inhibitors isolated from Brazilian plants: synthetic and natural molecules. BioMed Res Int 2013; 2013: 153045.
        [http://dx.doi.org/10.1155/2013/153045] [PMID: 24171158]

[6]   Benarba B, Meddah B. Ethnobotanical study, antifungal activity, phytochemical screening and total phenolic content of Algerian *Aristolochia longa.* J Intercult Ethnopharmacol 2014; 3(4) (Suppl.): 150-4.
        [http://dx.doi.org/10.5455/jice.20140826030222] [PMID: 26401365]

[7]   Dhouioui M, Boulilaa A, Chaabanea H, *et al.* Seasonal changes in essential oil composition of *Aristolochia longa* L ssp paucinervis Batt (*Aristolochiaceae*) roots and its antimicrobial activity. Ind Crops Prod 2016; 83: 301-6.
        [http://dx.doi.org/10.1016/j.indcrop.2016.01.025]

[8]   El Omari N, Sayah K, Fettach S, *et al.* Evaluation of *in vitro* antioxidant and antidiabetic activities of *Aristolochia longa* extracts. Evid Based Complement Alternat Med 2019; 2019: 9.
        [http://dx.doi.org/10.1155/2019/7384735]

[9]   El Yahyaoui El idrissi A, Talbaoui A, Bouyahya A, *et al.* Ethnobotanical study on the Bereztem Plant (*Aristolochia longa*) used in the treatment of some diseases in the cities of Rabat, Sale and Temara (Morocco). J Mater Environ Sci 2018; 9(6, suppl): 1914-21.

[10]   Aneb M, Talbaoui A, Bouyahya A, *et al. In vitro* cytotoxic effects and antibacterial activity of Moroccan medicinal plants *Aristolochia longa* and *Lavandula multifida.* EJMPl 2016; 16(2) (Suppl.): 1-13.
        [http://dx.doi.org/10.9734/EJMP/2016/28534]

[11]   Merouani N, Belhattab R, Sahli F. Evaluation of the biological activity of *Aristolochia longa* L. extracts. IJPSR 2017; 8(5) (Suppl.): 1978-92.

[12]   Benzakour G, Benkirane N, Amrani M, *et al.* Immunostimulatory potential of *Aristolochia longa* L. induced toxicity on liver, intestine and kidney in mice. J Toxicol Environ Health Sci 2011; 3(8) (Suppl.): 214-22.

[13]   Benzakour G, Amrani M, Oudghiri M. A Histopathological analyses of *in vivo* anti-tumor effect of an aqueous extract of *Aristolochia longa* used in cancer treatment in traditional medicine in Morocco. Int J Plant Res 2012; 2(2) (Suppl.): 31-5.
[http://dx.doi.org/10.5923/j.plant.20120202.06]

[14]   Benarba B, Pandiella A, Elmallah A. Anticancer activity, phytochemical screening and acute toxicity evaluation of an aqueous extract of *Aristolochia longa* L. Int J Pharm Phytopharm Res 2016; 20-6.

[15]   Cherif HS, Saidi F, Lazouri H, *et al.* Determination of the lipid compounds of *Aristolochia longa* L. from Algeria. Bulletin UASMV Agriculture 2009; 66(1) (Suppl.): 17-23.

[16]   Coste A. 3193 *Aristolochia longa* Tela botanica 2011. www.tela-botanica.org/bdtfx-nn-6468

[17]   Daoudi A, Bchiri L, Bammou M, *et al.* Etude ethnobotanique au Moyen Atlas Central. ESJ 2015; 11(24) (Suppl.): 1857-7881.

[18]   Salhi S, Fadli M, Zidane L, *et al.* Etudes floristique et ethnobotanique des plantes médicinales de la ville de Kénitra (Maroc). Lazaroa 2010; 31: 133-46.
[http://dx.doi.org/10.5209/rev_LAZA.2010.v31.9]

[19]   Bammi J, Allal D. Les plantes médicinales dans la forêt de l'Achach (Plateau Central, Maroc). ABM 2002; 27: 131-45.
[http://dx.doi.org/10.24310/abm.v27i0.7322]

[20]   Lahsissene H, Kahouadji A, Tijane M, *et al.* Catalogue des plantes médicinales utilisées dans la région de Zaër (Maroc Occidental). Lejeunia 2009; 186: 1-27.

[21]   Rhattas M, Allal D, Zidane L. Etude ethnobotanique des plantes médicinales dans le Parc National de Talassemtane (Rif Occidental du Maroc). J Appl Biosci 2016; 97: 9187-211.
[http://dx.doi.org/10.4314/jab.v97i1.5]

[22]   El-Hilaly J, Hmammouchi M, Lyoussi B. Ethnobotanical studies and economic evaluation of medicinal plants in Taounate province (Northern Morocco). J Ethnopharmacol 2003; 86(2-3): 149-58.
[http://dx.doi.org/10.1016/S0378-8741(03)00012-6] [PMID: 12738079]

[23]   Ghourri M, Lahcen Z, Allal D. Usage des plantes médicinales dans le traitement du diabète au Sahara marocain (Tan-Tan). J Anim Plant Sci 2013; 17: 2388-411.

[24]   W.H.O.. IARC Monographs on the Evaluation of Carcinogenic Risks to Humans: Some traditional herbal medicines, some mycotoxins, naphthalene and styrene. Lyon France: IARCPress 2002. No. 82.

[25]   Dauncey EA, Larsson S. Plants that kill: A Natural history of the world's most poisonous plants hardcover. Princeton, New Jersey: Princeton University Press 2018; p. 224.

[26]   Benarba B. Use of medicinal plants by breast cancer patients in Algeria. EXCLI J 2015; 14: 1164-6.
[PMID: 26713086]

[27]   Djeridane A, Yousfi M, Nadjemi B, Maamri S, Djireb F, Stocker P. Phenolic extracts from various Algerian plants as strong inhibitors of porcine liver carboxylesterase. J Enzyme Inhib Med Chem 2006; 21(6) (Suppl.): 719-26.
[http://dx.doi.org/10.1080/14756360600810399] [PMID: 17252945]

[28]   Cherif HS, Saidi F, Boutoumi H, *et al.* Identification et caracterisation de quelques composes chimiques chez *Aristolochia longa* L. Agricultura Ştiință şi practică 2009; 3(4, suppl): 71-2.

[29]   Ferreira ML, de Pascoli IC, Nascimento IR, Zukerman-Schpector J, Lopes LM. Aporphine and bisaporphine alkaloids from *Aristolochia lagesiana* var. intermedia. Phytochemistry 2010; 71(4) (Suppl.): 469-78.
[http://dx.doi.org/10.1016/j.phytochem.2009.11.010] [PMID: 20036405]

[30]   Machado MB, Lopes LMX. Tetraflavonoid and biflavonoids from *Aristolochia ridicula*. Phytochemistry 2008; 69(18) (Suppl.): 3095-102.
[http://dx.doi.org/10.1016/j.phytochem.2008.04.025] [PMID: 18561961]

[31]   Huang TC, Chen SM, Li YC, Lee JA. Increased renal semicarbazide-sensitive amine oxidase activity and methylglyoxal levels in aristolochic acid-induced nephrotoxicity. Life Sci 2014; 114(1) (Suppl.): 4-11.
[http://dx.doi.org/10.1016/j.lfs.2014.07.034] [PMID: 25107330]

[32]   Teresa JDP, Urones JG, Fernandez A. An aristolochic acid derivative from *Aristolochia longa.* Phytochemistry 1983; 22(12) (Suppl.): 2745-7.
[http://dx.doi.org/10.1016/S0031-9422(00)97687-8]

[33]   Shafi PM, Rosamma MK, Jamil K, Reddy PS. Antibacterial activity of the essential oil from *Aristolochia indica.* Fitoterapia 2002; 73(5): 439-41.
[http://dx.doi.org/10.1016/S0367-326X(02)00130-2] [PMID: 12165346]

[34]   Calleja MA, Vieites JM, Montero-Meléndez T, *et al.* The antioxidant effect of β-caryophyllene protects rat liver from carbon tetrachloride-induced fibrosis by inhibiting hepatic stellate cell activation. Br J Nutr 2013; 109(3) (Suppl.): 394-401.
[http://dx.doi.org/10.1017/S0007114512001298] [PMID: 22717234]

[35]   Guo L, Wu JZ, Han T, Cao T, Rahman K, Qin LP. Chemical composition, antifungal and antitumor properties of ether extracts of *Scapania verrucosa* Heeg. and its endophytic fungus *Chaetomium fusiforme.* Molecules 2008; 13(9) (Suppl.): 2114-25.
[http://dx.doi.org/10.3390/molecules13092114] [PMID: 18830144]

[36]   Rufino AT, Ribeiro M, Sousa C, *et al.* Evaluation of the anti-inflammatory, anti-catabolic and pro-anabolic effects of E-caryophyllene, myrcene and limonene in a cell model of osteoarthritis. Eur J Pharmacol 2015; 750: 141-50.
[http://dx.doi.org/10.1016/j.ejphar.2015.01.018] [PMID: 25622554]

[37]   Gupta CR. Nutraceuticals: Efficacy, safety and toxicity. 1st ed. Cambridge, Massachusetts: Elsevier 2016; pp. 735-60.

[38]   Pennathur S, Maitra D, Byun J, *et al.* Potent antioxidative activity of lycopene: A potential role in scavenging hypochlorous acid. Free Radic Biol Med 2010-15; 49(2, suppl): 205-13.
[http://dx.doi.org/10.1016/j.freeradbiomed.2010.04.003]

[39]   Hassan RA, Sand MI, El-Kadi MSh. Effect of some organic acids on fungal growth and their toxins production. J Agric Chem and Biotechn 2012; 3(9) (Suppl.): 391-7.
[http://dx.doi.org/10.21608/jacb.2012.55011]

[40]   Ryssel H, Kloeters O, Germann G, Schäfer T, Wiedemann G, Oehlbauer M. The antimicrobial effect of acetic acid--an alternative to common local antiseptics? Burns 2009; 35(5) (Suppl.): 695-700.
[http://dx.doi.org/10.1016/j.burns.2008.11.009] [PMID: 19286325]

[41]   Chen H, Chen T, Giudici P, *et al.* Vinegar functions on health: Constituents, sources, and formation mechanisms. CRFSFS 2016; 15(6) (Suppl.): 1124-38.
[http://dx.doi.org/10.1111/1541-4337.12228]

[42]   Trujillo WA, Sorenson WR, La Luzerne P, Austad JW, Sullivan D. Determination of aristolochic acid in botanicals and dietary supplements by liquid chromatography with ultraviolet detection and by liquid chromatography/mass spectrometry: single laboratory validation confirmation. J AOAC Int 2006; 89(4) (Suppl.): 942-59.
[http://dx.doi.org/10.1093/jaoac/89.4.942] [PMID: 16915829]

[43]   Abdelgadir AA, Ahmed EM, Eltohami MS. Isolation, characterization and quantity determination of aristolochic acids, toxic compounds in *Aristolochia bracteolata* L. Environ Health Insights 2011; 5: 1-8.
[http://dx.doi.org/10.4137/EHI.S6292] [PMID: 21487531]

[44]   Michl J, Ingrouille MJ, Simmonds MS, Heinrich M. Naturally occurring aristolochic acid analogues and their toxicities. Nat Prod Rep 2014; 31(5): 676-93.
[http://dx.doi.org/10.1039/c3np70114j] [PMID: 24691743]

[45] Dhouioui M, Boulila A, Jemli M, Schiets F, Casabianca H, Zina MS. Fatty acids composition and antibacterial activity of *Aristolochia longa* L. and *Bryonia dioïca* Jacq. Growing wild in Tunisia. J Oleo Sci 2016; 65(8) (Suppl.): 655-61.
[http://dx.doi.org/10.5650/jos.ess16001] [PMID: 27430383]

[46] Harada H, Yamashita U, Kurihara H, Fukushi E, Kawabata J, Kamei Y. Antitumor activity of palmitic acid found as a selective cytotoxic substance in a marine red alga. Anticancer Res 2002; 22(5) (Suppl.): 2587-90.
[PMID: 12529968]

[47] Zheng CJ, Yoo JS, Lee TG, Cho HY, Kim YH, Kim WG. Fatty acid synthesis is a target for antibacterial activity of unsaturated fatty acids. FEBS Lett 2005; 579(23) (Suppl.): 5157-62.
[http://dx.doi.org/10.1016/j.febslet.2005.08.028] [PMID: 16146629]

[48] Singh S, Nair V, Jain S, Gupta YK. Evaluation of anti-inflammatory activity of plant lipids containing α-linolenic acid. Indian J Exp Biol 2008; 46(6) (Suppl.): 453-6.
[PMID: 18697604]

[49] Calde PC. Mechanisms of action of (n-3) fatty fcids. J Nutr 2012; 142(3) (Suppl.): 592-9.
[http://dx.doi.org/10.3945/jn.111.155259]

[50] Yoon BK, Jackman JA, Valle-González ER, Cho NJ. Antibacterial free fatty acids and monoglycerides: Biological activities, experimental testing and therapeutic applications. Int J Mol Sci 2018; 19(4) (Suppl.): 1114.
[http://dx.doi.org/10.3390/ijms19041114] [PMID: 29642500]

[51] Legault J, Pichette A. Potentiating effect of β-caryophyllene on anticancer activity of α-humulene, isocaryophyllene and paclitaxel. J Pharm Pharmacol 2007; 59(12) (Suppl.): 1643-7.
[http://dx.doi.org/10.1211/jpp.59.12.0005] [PMID: 18053325]

[52] Belosludtsev K, Saris NE, Andersson LC, *et al.* On the mechanism of palmitic acid-induced apoptosis: the role of a pore induced by palmitic acid and Ca^{2+} in mitochondria. J Bioenerg Biomembr 2006; 38(2): 113-20.
[http://dx.doi.org/10.1007/s10863-006-9010-9] [PMID: 16847595]

[53] Alves-Silva JM, Romane A, Efferth T, Salgueiro L. North african medicinal plants traditionally used in cancer therapy. Front Pharmacol 2017; 8: 383.
[http://dx.doi.org/10.3389/fphar.2017.00383] [PMID: 28694778]

[54] Hinou J, Demetzos C, Harvala C, *et al.* Cytotoxic and antimicrobial arinciples from the roots of *Aristolochia longa*. Int J Crude Drug Res 1990; 28(2) (Suppl.): 149-51.
[http://dx.doi.org/10.3109/13880209009082801]

[55] Arlt VM, Stiborová M, vom Brocke J, *et al.* Aristolochic acid mutagenesis: molecular clues to the aetiology of Balkan endemic nephropathy-associated urothelial cancer. Carcinogenesis 2007; 28(11): 2253-61.
[http://dx.doi.org/10.1093/carcin/bgm082] [PMID: 17434925]

[56] Pozdzik AA, Berton A, Schmeiser HH, *et al.* Aristolochic acid nephropathy revisited: a place for innate and adaptive immunity? Histopathology 2010; 56(4) (Suppl.): 449-63.
[http://dx.doi.org/10.1111/j.1365-2559.2010.03509.x] [PMID: 20459552]

[57] Benarba B, Meddah M, Tir Touil A. Response of bone resorption markers to *Aristolochia longa* intake by Algerian breast cancer postmenopausal women. Adv Pharmacol Sci 2014; 2014: 820589.

[58] Bouyahya A, Bakri Y, Khay EO, *et al.* Antibacterial, antioxidant and anti-tumor properties of Moroccan medicinal plants: A review. Asian Pac J Trop Dis 2017; 7(1): 57-64.
[http://dx.doi.org/10.12980/apjtd.7.2017D6-294]

[59] Hajji H, Talbaoui A, Faris Elalaoui FE, *et al. In vitro* evaluation of antibacterial action of *Caralluma europaea* extracts on *Rhodococcus equi*. J Chem Pharm Res 2016; 8(5) (Suppl.): 943-52.

[60]   Girija S, Duraipandiyan V, Kuppusamy PS, *et al.* Chromatographic characterization and GC-MS evaluation of the bioactive constituents with antimicrobial potential from the pigmented Ink of *Loligo duvauceli.* ISRN 2014; 2014: pp. 1-7.

[61]   Preedy V, Watson R. Olives and olive oil in health and disease prevention. Cambridge, Massachusetts: Academic Press 2010; pp. 1283-8.

[62]   Karan SK, Mishra SK, Pal D, *et al.* Isolation of *β*-sitosterol and evaluation of antidiabetic activity of *Aristolochia indica* in alloxan-induced diabetic mice with a reference to *in vitro* antioxidant activity. JMPR 2012; 6(7) (Suppl.): 1219-23.

[63]   Adefegha SA, Oboh G. *In vitro* inhibition activity of polyphenol-rich extracts from *Syzygium aromaticum* (L.) Merr. & Perry (Clove) buds against carbohydrate hydrolyzing enzymes linked to type 2 diabetes and $Fe^{(2+)}$ induced lipid peroxidation in rat pancreas. Asian Pac J Trop Biomed 2012; 2(10) (Suppl.): 774-81.
[http://dx.doi.org/10.1016/S2221-1691(12)60228-7] [PMID: 23569846]

[64]   Basha RH, Sankaranarayanan C. β-Caryophyllene, a natural sesquiterpene, modulates carbohydrate metabolism in streptozotocin-induced diabetic rats. Acta Histochem 2014; 116(8) (Suppl.): 1469-79.
[http://dx.doi.org/10.1016/j.acthis.2014.10.001] [PMID: 25457874]

[65]   Badami S, Jose CK, Kumar CRK, *et al. In vitro* antioxidant activity of various extracts of *Aristolochia bracteolata* leaves. Orient Pharm Exp Med 2005; 5(4) (Suppl.): 316-21.
[http://dx.doi.org/10.3742/OPEM.2005.5.4.316]

[66]   Derouiche S, Zeghib K, Gharbi S, *et al.* Beneficial effects of *Aristolochia longa* and *Aquilaria malaccensis* on Lead-Induced hematological alterations and heart oxidative stress in rats. J Chem Pharm Res 2018; 10(9) (Suppl.): 8-15.

[67]   Dipasquale D, Basiricò L, Morera P, Primi R, Tröscher A, Bernabucci U. Anti-inflammatory effects of conjugated linoleic acid isomers and essential fatty acids in bovine mammary epithelial cells. Animal 2018; 12(10) (Suppl.): 2108-14.
[http://dx.doi.org/10.1017/S1751731117003676] [PMID: 29310736]

[68]   Houghton P. Anti-inflammatory plants ethnopharmacology of medicinal plants: Asia and the pacific. Br J Clin Pharmacol 2007; 64(2) (Suppl.): 248.

[69]   Delves TJ, Roitt IM. Encyclopedia of immunology. 2nd ed. London: Academic Press 1998; pp. 198-231.

[70]   Raphael TJ, Kuttan G. Effect of naturally occurring triterpenoids glycyrrhizic acid, ursolic acid, oleanolic acid and nomilin on the immune system. Phytomedicine 2003; 10(6-7): 483-9.
[http://dx.doi.org/10.1078/094471103322331421] [PMID: 13678231]

[71]   Derouiche S, Zeghib K, Gharbi S, *et al.* Protective effects of *Aristolochia longa* and *Aquilaria malaccensis* against lead induced acute liver injury in rats. J Acute Dis 2017; 6(5) (Suppl.): 193-7.
[http://dx.doi.org/10.4103/2221-6189.219611]

[72]   Jackson L, Kofman S, Weiss A, Brodovsky H. Aristolochic acid (NSC-50413): Phase I clinical study. Cancer Chemother Rep 1964; 42: 35-7.
[PMID: 14226128]

CHAPTER 9

Wound Healing Potential of Combined Extracts of Stem Bark and Leaves of *Sphenocentrum Jollyanum*: A Classical Factorial Design Model Approach

Charles O. Nnadi[1,*], Chinwe M. Onah[1], Chigozie L. Ugwu[2] and Wilfred O. Obonga[1]

[1] *Department of Pharmaceutical and Medicinal Chemistry, Faculty of Pharmaceutical Sciences, University of Nigeria Nsukka, 410001 Nsukka, Nigeria*

[2] *Department of Statistics, Faculty of Physical Sciences, University of Nigeria Nsukka, 410001 Nsukka, Nigeria*

Abstract: Stem bark, in combination with the leaves of *Sphenocentrum jollyanum*, is used for the management of wounds in the Southern part of Nigeria. The wound healing potential was determined by applying different concentrations of the prepared plant extracts, alone and in combination, to deep partial-thickness wounds on a rat model. Wound healing was measured on 15 days post-operation and compared with the controls. The percentage wound closure efficacy of the combined leaves and stem bark extracts were determined and compared statistically by 2^2 Factorial design model over 2, 8, and 15 post-operative days. Fluctuations in the wound surface pH were also measured over 15 days. All the extracts-treated wounds epithelized faster with dose-dependent wound contraction, reaching statistically significant differences ($p<0.01$) compared with untreated wounds. The stem bark extract was about 50% more potent than the leaves extract. A significantly higher wound contraction effect of combined extracts was observed when compared with the individual extract effects. Also interesting was the <10 days complete epithelization observed in combined (200 mg equivalent) leaves and stem bark-treated wounds, which is shorter than 13 post-operative days in both 100 mg stem bark extract- and cicatrin-treated groups. However, there was no statistical evidence (*$p<0.0$) of interaction between the leaves and stem bark extracts; and improved activities of the combined extracts, in comparison with the individual extracts, were purely additive. The initial alkaline wound surface pH normalized to acidic pH within 8 and 12 post-operative days in extracts- and positive control-treated wounds. *S. jollyanum* extracts possess promising wound healing property. This study validated the primary folkloric use of the plant and aside from additive effect, empirical and statistical evidences showed that there was no basis for the claimed potency of combined leaves and stem as used by the traditional healers.

* **Corresponding author Charles O. Nnadi:** Department of Pharmaceutical and Medicinal Chemistry, Faculty of Pharmaceutical Sciences, University of Nigeria Nsukka, 410001 Nsukka, Nigeria; Tel: +2348 0649 47734; E-mail: charles.nnadi@unn.edu.ng

Anna Capasso (Ed.)

Keywords: Ethnomedicine, Factorial design, *Sphenocentrum jollyanum*, Wound contraction.

INTRODUCTION

The global burden of wound management is enormous, considering the level of illness, prolonged hospital stay, potential disability, excess costs, and sometimes death resulting from untreated wounds [1]. About 15.3 billion USD was projected to be spent annually on wound care products in the US alone by 2010 [2]; the estimate was overwhelmed at 25 billion USD was spent in 2016 alone to treat wound-related complications [3]. The situation is more disturbing in developing countries as the challenges, in terms of mortality and morbidity [4], are usually complicated by unaffordable sophisticated remedy. In Nigeria, for instance, many people still rely on medicinal plant products for the management of wounds and other ailments due to their availability, efficacy, presumed safety, and affordability [5, 6]. *Sphenocentrum jollyanum* Pierre (family Menispermaceae) is a wild tropical plant commonly distributed in Nigeria and other West African countries [7]. The plant is used traditionally in Nigeria as chewing stick, aphrodisiac and also as a remedy for cough, fever and chronic wounds [8 - 10]. Previous studies showed that various morphological parts have antipyretic, analgesic, anti-inflammatory, antioxidant, antidiabetic [11 - 15], antimalarial [16], steroidogenic, and antifatigue [17] activities. Its activity against the Polio Type-2 virus has also been documented [13]. In Nigeria, the plant is locally called Ezeogwu (king of herbs) or Orji-nkoro in Igbo, Oban Abe in Edo and Akerejupon in Yoruba languages and has been claimed to possess wound healing activity [9], which is yet to be validated. This claim has been sustained in Southern Nigeria by the African traditional and complementary medicine (ATCM) practitioners due to its ethnotherapeutic potency. These traditional healers claimed, in addition, that its wound healing property is evidenced only when both the leaves and stem bark are ground together with few drops of water and the squeezed pulp from the paste is applied to fresh wounds.

The validity or otherwise of these claims is still unknown. This study, therefore, seeks to (i) investigate separately the wound healing properties of the aqueous extracts of stem bark and leaves, and further (ii) determine the wound healing potential of these combined aqueous extracts with the objective of validating the folkloric claims of the herbal uses of *S. jollyanum* leaves and stem bark.

MATERIALS AND METHODS

Collection and Processing of Plant Materials

The plant materials (fresh stem bark and leaves) were collected in 2018 with the help of a traditional healer from a forest in Benue State Nigeria (N 7 43' 50", E 8 32' 10"); and identified and authenticated by a taxonomist at the Institute of Plant Science and Biotechnology, University of Nigeria Nsukka. A voucher specimen (UNH 302m) was prepared and stored at the herbarium of the Institute for future reference. The plant name was further confirmed at http://www.theplantlist.org on 20th December 2018.

Preparation of The Plant Extracts

The plant extracts were prepared in line with the ethno-pharmacological information obtained from ATCM practitioners and local users. A 1000 g each of the fresh plant materials was washed with distilled water and allowed to drain completely under the shade. The plant materials were pulverized and the extract was squeezed with fresh distilled water. The mixture was filtered thereafter and the filtrates were concentrated to dryness by freeze-drying. The dried extracts were preserved at 4 °C until use. The application of the plant extracts was also done according to the traditional healers' instructions by placing directly on the fresh wounds as described subsequently.

Phytochemical Analysis of Plant Extracts

The crude extracts of *S. jollyanum* were tested for the presence or absence of major secondary metabolites such as glycosides, saponins, anthraquinones, flavonoids, terpenoids, tannins, alkaloids, and reducing the sugar by standard method [18]. Quantification of secondary metabolites in both extracts was performed by standardized methods [18 - 21].

Experimental Animals and Test Groups

Albino rats (±50 g) of either sex were used for the excision wound healing study and were divided into treatment groups of five rats each, as described below. All the experimental animals were acclimatized for 14 days, with free access to standard animal feed and water, distinctively marked and weighed prior to the study. All the animals were handled in line with the University of Nigeria Ethics Committee guidelines on the handling of laboratory animals and other related products.

Surgical Infliction of Excision Wound

The rats were anesthetized using injectable ketamine hydrochloride, 5 mg/kg, i.v (Supriya Lifescience Ltd., India). The wounds of about 400 mm^2 circular area and 2 mm depth were inflicted on each rat by a veterinary surgeon, following previously reported protocols [22]. The wounds were left open to the environment for 12 h before initiation of treatment.

Wound Treatment

Prior to the treatment of the wounds, the plant extracts were moistened with an equal volume of distilled water in the form that would adhere to the wounds. The wounds were thereafter treated with one of the following: (a) 0.5 ml distilled water as a negative control, Group I; (b) 20, 50, and 100 mg of prepared stem bark extract for Groups IIa, IIb, and IIc, respectively; (c) 20, 50, and 100 mg of prepared leaves extract for Groups IIIa, IIIb and IIIc, respectively; (d) 40, 100, and 200 mg of combined stem bark and leaves extracts (1:1) for Groups IVa, Ivb, and Ivc, respectively; or (e) 50 mg cicatrin (GSK Pakistan Ltd, Karachi), a commercially available neomycin sulphate and bacitracin zinc combination, as a positive control, Group V. Each treated wound was covered with a dressing containing absorptive pad. The animals were properly marked and housed in the Animal Unit, with free access to their normal diets. The concentrations of the extracts in the prepared samples applied to the wounds were determined based on the preliminary wound healing investigations and pilot study. The wounds were cleaned daily with dilute (1:100) Dettol antiseptic (Reckitt Benckiser Ltd, Nigeria) to prevent possible microbial infection and various treatments were applied once daily for 15 days.

Data Collection and Analysis

The wound area was measured on 0, 2, 4, 8, 12, and 15 post-operative days and until healing was complete. The epithelization times (number of days taken for complete wound closure and falling off of dead tissue remnants) were recorded. The percentages of excision wound closure (with respect to the initial wound areas) were calculated. On day 0 and prior to wound cleaning on post-operative days 2, 4, 8, 12 and 15, the wounds surface pH of Groups I, IIc, IIIc, Ivc, and V were measured and their profiles were plotted accordingly.

Statistical Analysis

The experimental results were analyzed using the Statistical Package for the Social Sciences (SPSS Inc. Chicago), v. 15.0 and GraphPad Prism v. 6.01.2012 (GraphPad Software Inc., San Diego, CA, USA) software. The excision wound areas were expressed as a mean ± standard error of the mean (SEM) (n=5). One way analysis of variance (ANOVA) was done to test for the significant difference between the means of samples and control at $p<0.01$ by post-hoc using 2-sided Dunnett's test. In all cases, $p < 0.01$ was considered to be significant.

To determine the overall effect of combined stem bark and leaves extract on wound closure, a factorial design statistical model was used to compare the differences between means of samples and negative control [23]. The two factors (leaves and stem extracts) were considered at the two extreme concentration levels (20 and 100 mg) applied on the wound and 40 and 200 mg combined extracts (1:1) to determine the additivity or interactivity of the leaves and stem extracts to the wound healing activity. In all levels of the factors, the effect of one factor in the combination was calculated as the summation of the mean effect of the factor alone less than that of the negative control and combined effect less than the effect of complementary factor alone. In all cases, a $*p<0$ was considered the additive effect of the factors and a $*p>0$ as an interaction of factors.

RESULTS

Phytochemical Constituents of Plant Extracts

Phytochemical analysis showed similarity in the composition of secondary metabolites in the stem and leaves extracts of *S. jollyanum*. Alkaloid, saponins, anthraquinones, flavonoids, tannins, and reducing sugar were detected in the leaves and stem bark extracts, as shown in Table **1**. A higher amount of tannin was detected in the leaves, while the stem extract was alkaloid-rich with a composition of 13.5 g/100g. Cardiac glycoside was not detected in the stem bark, with a trace amount contained in the leaves extract. The absence of terpenoids in both extracts could be attributed to the extracting solvent's inability to extract non-polar constituents; its presence otherwise can only be confirmed when methanol or less polar solvent is used for the extraction.

Table 1. Phytochemical composition of extracts of *Sphenocentrum jollyanum*..

Secondary Metabolites	Composition (Mg/100 g)	
	Stem Bark Extract	Leaves Extract
Alkaloids	13.58±0.92	8.04±0.21

(Table 1) cont.....

Anthroquinones	0.90±0.11	2.94±0.05
Flavonoids	1.92±0.20	3.05±0.82
Reducing sugars	4.06±0.01	1.19±0.04
Saponin	2.50±0.03	3.02±0.72
Tannins	7.82±0.62	16.01±1.10
Cardiac glycosides	-	Trace
Terpenoids	-	-
Phenolics	5.01±0.12	3.52±1.01

Wound Closure Effects of Plant Extracts

The excision wound areas measured over 15 days post-operation and the epithelization times were recorded in Table 2. The wound closure was generally dose-dependent. Higher wound healing efficacy and shorter epithelization time were observed in stem bark extracts compared with the leaves at the same dose levels. All applied doses of stem bark extracts showed a statistically significant difference in wound healing effects ($p < 0.01$) compared with the negative control over 15 days. Similar results were observed when compared with the positive control, with the exception of 50 mg dose on the 15th day and 100 mg dose on the 2nd, 4th, 12th, and 15th post-operative days. When compared with the combined effects of leaves and stem bark extracts, there were no statistically significant differences ($p>0.01$) in the wound healing efficacies except for 20 mg applied dose on day 2, and 100 mg dose on days 2, 4, and 8 post-operative. Complete healing time was shortest for high doses of combined extracts, more than 4 days compared with the positive control. When compared dose-to-dose effects, the combined extracts were more potent than the stem bark extracts alone, reaching a statistically significant difference ($p < 0.01$) with the positive control over 4 days (40 and 100 mg), 8 days (40 mg), and 12 days (40 mg) post-operative. However, the epithelization was completed in lesser time.

Table 2. Effects of extracts of *S. jollyanum* on excision wound model in rats.

Group	Post-Operative Days/ Wound Area (MM²)						Epithelization (days)
	0	2	4	8	12	15	
I	405.2±4.8	400.8±4.7	394.2±4.3	332.8±17.0	256.4±23.6	224.8±15.0	24.8±1.6
IIa	400.4±2.6	315.2±5.8[abc]	210.2±8.1[ac]	136.4±52.0[ac]	44.8±3.9[ac]	32.4±2.6[ac]	16.6±0.9
IIb	400.0±6.5	300.0±6.5[ac]	202.2±3.3[ac]	118.8±20.1[ac]	38.0±5.5[ac]	4.4±2.6[a]	16.4±0.5
IIc	400.8±5.8	296.0±5.7[ab]	189.2±6.7[ab]	95.2±4.1[abc]	12.6±2.8[a]	0.0±0.0[a]	13.6±0.5
IIIa	407.4±8.2	360.0±12.7[abc]	327.6±6.1[abc]	287.2±8.8[abc]	218.8±9.4[abc]	184.8±3.6[abc]	21.6±1.1
IIIb	402.8±5.4	334.4±5.2[abc]	259.2±19.3[abc]	208.4±8.5[abc]	157,6±7.8[abc]	120.0±15.8[abc]	18.2±1.3

(Table 2) cont.....

IIIc	401.2±5.4	319.2±7.3[abc]	240.0±8.2[abc]	194.8±6.7[abc]	136.8±9.9[abc]	103.6±4.3[abc]	17.8±0.4
IVa	403.0±3.2	298.0±14.8[a]	201.6±2.6[ac]	116.0±20.1[ac]	36.2±2.9[ac]	4.8±2.3[a]	16.2±0.4
IVb	400.8±7.8[a]	295.2±5.8[a]	168.0±22.8[ac]	14.8±3.9[a]	1.4±1.3[a]	0.0±0.0[a]	13.0±0.7
IVc	401.4±7.3[a]	250.0±15.8[a]	149.6±7.4[a]	26.4±4.8[a]	0.0±0.0[a]	0.0±0.0[a]	9.8±0.8
V	401.4±1.7	265.6±11.3	165.2±11.2	49.2±7.3	4.8±2.3	0.0±0.0	13.0±0.7

Results are expressed as mean ± SEM (n=5); $p < 0.01$ ascompared with [a]negative control, [b]combined leaves and stem extracts, and [c]positive control. One way ANOVA followed by Dunett t-test, 2-sided.

Effects of Combined Extracts on Wound Healing Activities

The actual contribution of each of the leaves and stem bark to the overall combined wound closure effect was established by a 2^2 factorial design model (Table **3**). Each of the extracts contributed less to the overall effects of the combined extracts in comparison with the individual effects when applied alone on fresh wounds. When 20 mg extracts were applied separately, a 32.9% empirical additive wound closure was evident on day 2 post-operative as against 25.6% obtained from factorial design statistical approach. This statistical effect was also found to be slightly lower than the actual empirical additive wound closure effect (26.13%) of the combined leaves and stem bark (data shown on Supplementary file, Fig. **2**) recorded when 40 mg combined extracts (1:1) was applied on day 2 post-operative. Similar observation was recorded for 100 mg applied extracts on the 15th day post-operative. There was no interaction recorded for the two factors, two levels at the day intervals considered.

Table 3. Interaction/ additive wound closure effects of combined extracts of *S. jollyanum..*

Days	Levels (mg)	Wound Healing Effects (%)					
		[a]SMEm	[a]LMEm	[b]SMEm in LSEm	[c]LME in LSEm	[d]additivity	[e]interaction
2	20	21.3±1.6	11.6±2.4	17.30	7.17	25.6*	-
	100	26.1±1.9	20.4±1.8	21.13	15.44	37.7±4.4	-
8	20	65.9±12.9	29.5±2.0	44.89	8.44	71.2±5.1	-
	100	76.3±0.7	51.4±1.5	50.16	25.35	93.4±1.3	-
15	20	91.9±0.6	54.6±1.1	45.78	8.50	98.8±0.6	-
	100	100±0.0	74.2±1.2	40.65	7.41	92.6*	-

[a]Data expressed as mean±SEM of wound healing (%) with respect to wound area on day 0, [b]actual effect of stem bark alone, SMEm in the combined extract, LSEm (calculated as the mean effect of SMEm alone less the negative control and LSEm less the effect of leaves extract alone, LMEm alone), [c]actual effect of LMEm in the combined extract (calculated as the mean effect of LMEm alone less the negative control and LSEm less the effect of SMEm alone), [d]values corresponds to statistical effect of LSEm, if merely additive, [e]calcualted as the mean difference of the effect of SMEm in the presence and absence of LMEm [23]; and considered as interaction if >0; additive, if otherwise.*slightly different from the actual values obtained for the combined effects.

Wound Surface pH Profile

The initial pH profile of the fresh wound was 7.65-7.88 units (Fig. **1**). Treatments led to pH surge 2 days post-operatively to 8.42 and 8.35 for negative and positive control groups, respectively, and to 8.03, 8.25, and 8.16 for stem, leaves, and combined extracts experimental groups, respectively. Thereafter, the decline in pH followed similar trends, with those of the experimental plant extracts normalizing within 8 days and positive controls 12 days post-operatively.

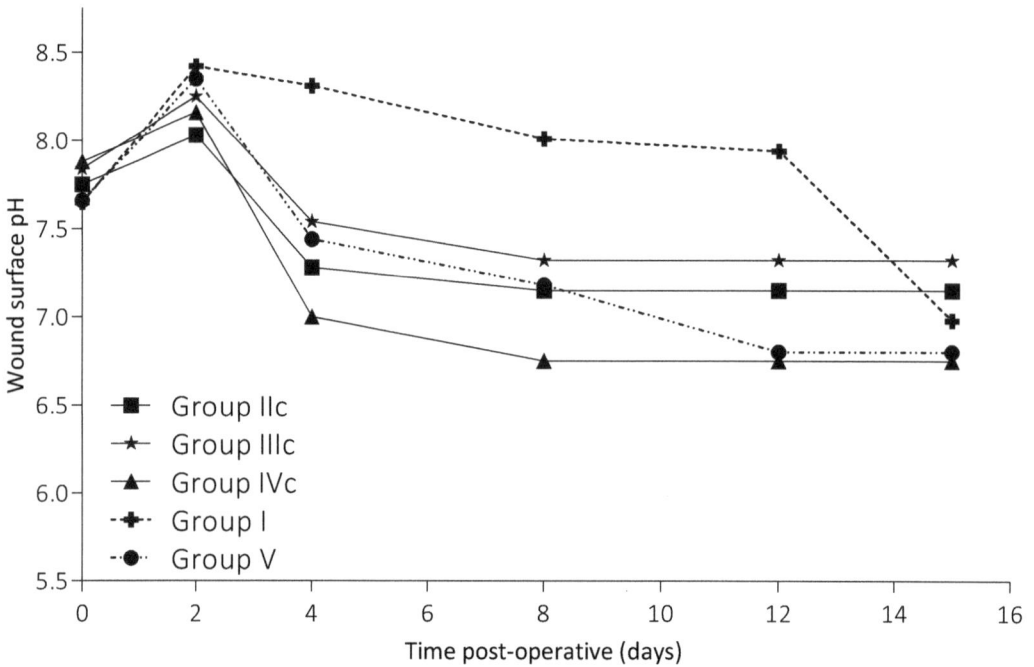

Fig. (1). Post-operative wound surface pH changes over 15 days.

DISCUSSION

Wound healing involves cascades of biochemical mechanisms to repair compromised skin [24]. Such mechanisms can be triggered by biochemical molecules, such as secondary metabolites or by the immune system, such as antibodies. This study identified the critical roles of *S. jollyanum* extracts prepared in line with the ethnopharmacological data in wound healing; and further confirmed that the combination of both extracts, as used by traditional healers, may not be necessary, thus complementing its anti-inflammatory, antioxidant, antiviral, and steroidogenic, antiparasitic, antipyretic, analgesic activities [11 - 17].

Interestingly, all the extract produced significant percentage wound closure effects (>11% for the leaves, >21% for stem bark and >26% for the combined extracts) within 2 days post-operative. This relative high wound contraction suggests that the plant extracts influence early phases of wound healing, such as accelerated proliferation and/or maturation of the epidermal layer. More so, the wound closure effects in the negative control groups could be attributed to the innate immune system of the animals. A factorial design model established a statistical additive wound closure of 25.6% on the 2nd day post-operative, slightly lower than 26.13% obtained from the empirical data on treatment with 20 mg equivalent each of the extract in combination. With an SEM of ±3.65%, this slight discrepancy was unaccounted for by this study but could also be attributed to rapid initiation of hemostasis stage and completed healing was observed before the 15th day post-operative. For the combined 100 mg stem bark and 100 mg leaves extract, the healing process was completed before the 10th post-operative day, suggesting that the individual contributions of the extracts to the overall wound closure and epithelization were merely additive. These were expected at least at later phases (maturation and remodeling) of the healing process when the individual extracts had no additional effect on the overall additive effect of the combined extracts. The interaction level calculated using the factorial design model showed values less than zero, indicating the absence of any form of interaction [23] between the wound contraction efficacies of the stem bark and leaves extracts. However, the stem bark extract contributed more than 50% wound healing activity at most of the applied doses during the treatment and healing days, an indication of the presence of more active secondary metabolites in the stem bark. Nevertheless, the significant healing activities recorded for each of the leaves and stem bark, when used separately, further confirmed that combining them, as advocated by the traditional healers, could be avoided without compromising the potency. Such claimed practices would have been meaningful if significant wound healing was not recorded when used alone and empirical or statistical data suggested significant interaction thereof.

Wound closure requires constant modulation of some growth factors, cytoplasmic receptor domains, and cytokines in addition to the removal of cellular debris [25, 26]. Appropriate pH of the intact mammalian skin maintains homeostasis and the correct balance of protease and promotes cell migration and proliferation, which are required for wound healing [27]. Typically, the pH changes of all the plant extracts- and cicatrin-treated wounds assumed four similar but distinct phases: (a) initial pH surge to alkaline, followed by (b) downturn towards neutrality, then (c) to acidity levels, and finally (d) normalization. However, the extracts-treated wounds normalized earlier than the cicatrin-treated. The implications of the observed distinct stages of wound healing in this study were not probed but this suggested possibility of a similar mechanism with cicatrin; however, biochemical changes in the various stages of wound healing [27] could be a plausible explanation for these. More so, whether the four distinct phases in wound surface pH are related to the four phases of wound healing—haemostasis, inflammation, proliferation, and remodeling- requires further analysis.

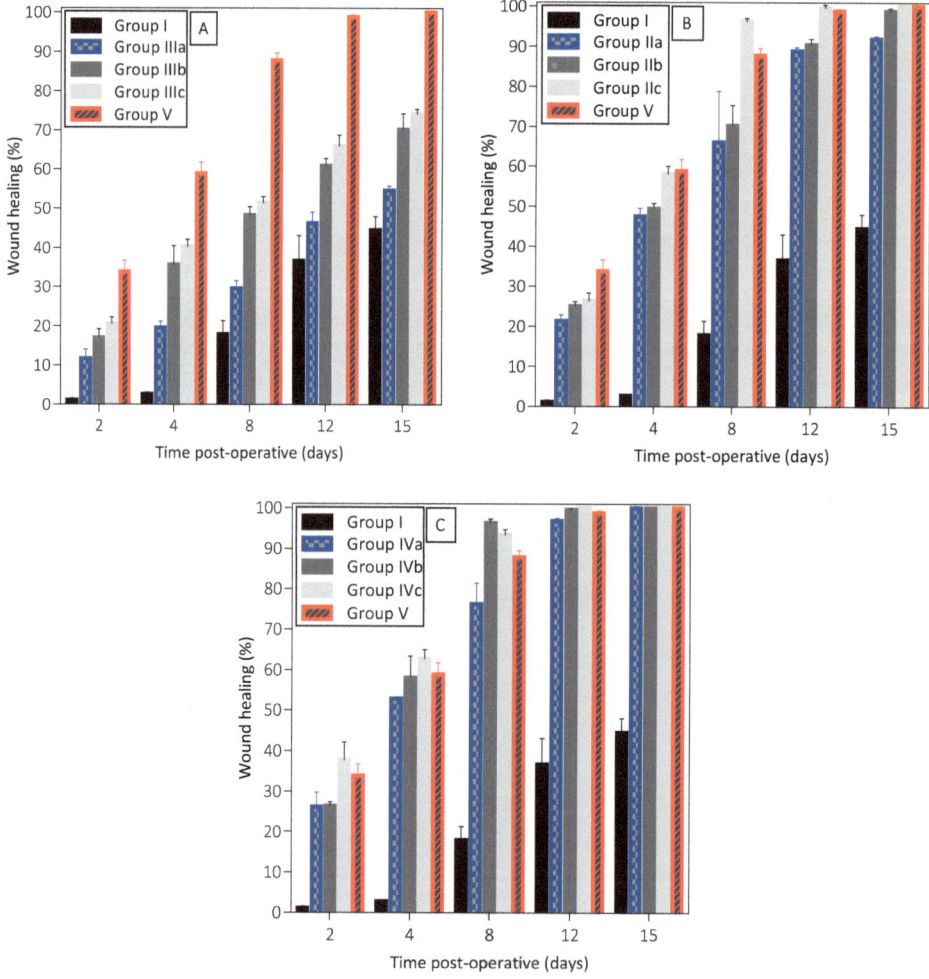

Fig. (2). Percentage wound closure efficacy of leaves **(A)**, stem bark **(B)** and combined leaves and stem bark **(C)** extracts of *S. jollyanum*.

In this study, therefore, it must be noted that the chemical composition or the concentration of the active principle(s) was unknown. However, phytochemical constituents of plants have been implicated in several biological activities of plants, including *S. jollyanum* [11 - 17, 28]. The major significant differences observed in this case were in the alkaloidal, tannins, and anthraquinone compositions, which have also been implicated elsewhere in the wound healing efficacy of plants [22, 29 - 33]. Interestingly, an alkaloid extracted from *Croton lechleri* was found to stimulate chemotaxis for fibroblasts [31, 34]. Similarly, anthraquinone-rich *Rheum officinale* was found to promote wound healing *via* a complex mechanism, involving tissue regeneration stimulation and regulation of other signaling pathways [33]. To confirm the connection of the present study with these findings, however, would require (i) isolation of the active compound(s); which is currently in progress, (ii) quantification of the compound responsible for wound healing for further optimization, (iii) determination of mechanism of wound healing activity, (iv) determination of topical toxicity profile and (v) formulation into suitable delivery form.

CONCLUSION

S. jollyanum leaves and stem bark extracts possess promising wound contraction activities. The impressive activity at doses <100 mg of the crude extract is worth investigating further. Interestingly, there was no interaction in the activities of both stem bark and leaves, though the stem bark extract-treated wounds epithelized faster than both the leaves extract and cicatrin-treated wounds. This has validated the ethnomedicinal use of the plant as a potential source of wound cicatrizant, on one hand, but could not support the rationale behind the claimed combination due to the obvious absence of interaction of activity.

CONSENT FOR PUBLICATION

Not Applicable.

CONFLICT OF INTEREST

The author declares no conflict of interest, financial or otherwise.

ACKNOWLEDGEMENTS

Declared none.

REFERENCES

[1]   Bagheri Nejad S, Allegranzi B, Syed SB, Ellis B, Pittet D. Health-care-associated infection in Africa: a systematic review. Bull World Health Organ 2011; 89(10): 757-65.
       [http://dx.doi.org/10.2471/BLT.11.088179] [PMID: 22084514]

[2]   Sen CK, Gordillo GM, Roy S, *et al.* Human skin wounds: a major and snowballing threat to public health and the economy. Wound Repair Regen 2009; 17(6): 763-71.
       [http://dx.doi.org/10.1111/j.1524-475X.2009.00543.x] [PMID: 19903300]

[3]   Järbrink K, Ni G, Sönnergren H, *et al.* The humanistic and economic burden of chronic wounds: a protocol for a systematic review. Syst Rev 2017; 6(1): 15.
       [http://dx.doi.org/10.1186/s13643-016-0400-8] [PMID: 28118847]

[4]   Murthy S, Gautam MK, Goel S, Purohit V, Sharma H, Goel RK. Evaluation of *in vivo* wound healing activity of *Bacopa monniera* on different wound model in rats. Biomed Res Int 2013; 9.
[http://dx.doi.org/10.1155/2013/972028] [PMID: 972028]

[5]   Gupta AK, Vats SK, Lal B. How cheap can a medicinal plant species be? Curr Sci 1998; 74(7): 565-6.

[6]   Caccia-Bava MDCGG, Bertoni BW, Pereira AMS, Martinez EZ. Availability of herbal medicines and medicinal plants in the primary health facilities of the state of São Paulo, Southeast Brazil: results from the National Program for Access and Quality Improvement in Primary Care. Cien Saude Colet 2017; 22(5): 1651-9.
[http://dx.doi.org/10.1590/1413-81232017225.16722015] [PMID: 28538934]

[7]   Nia R, Paper DH, Essien EE, *et al.* Evaluation of the antioxidant and antiangiogenic effects of *sphenocentrum jollyanum* Pierre. Afr J Biomed Res 2004; 7: 129-32.

[8]   Iwu MM. Handbook of African medicinal plants. Boca Raton: CRC Press Inc 1993.

[9]   Dalziel JM. The useful plants of West tropical Africa. London: Crown Agents 1937.

[10]   Irvine FR. Woody Plants of Ghana. London: Oxford University press 1961.

[11]   Mbaka G, Adeyemi O, Osinubi A, Noronha C, Okanlawon A. The effect of aqueous root extract of *Sphenocentrum jollyanum* on blood glucose level of rabbits. J Med Plants Res 2009; 3(11): 870-4.

[12]   Muko KN, Ohiri PC, Ezegwu CO. Antipyretic and analgesic activities of *Sphenocentrum jollyanum.* Niger J Nat Prod Med 1998; 2: 52-3.
[http://dx.doi.org/10.4314/njnpm.v2i1.11785]

[13]   Moody JO, Robberts VA, Adeniji JA. Antiviral effect of selected medicinal plants 1: effect of *Diospyros bateri, Diospyros monbutensis* and *Sphenocentrum jollyanum* on polio viruses. Niger J Nat Prod Med 2002; 6: 4-6.
[http://dx.doi.org/10.4314/njnpm.v6i1.11682]

[14]   Moody JO, Robert VA, Connolly JD, Houghton PJ. Anti-inflammatory activities of the methanol extracts and an isolated furanoditerpene constituent of *Sphenocentrum jollyanum* Pierre (Menispermaceae). J Ethnopharmacol 2006; 104(1-2): 87-91.
[http://dx.doi.org/10.1016/j.jep.2005.08.051] [PMID: 16236477]

[15]   Samuel FO, Sinbad OO, Olusoji O. In-vitro anti-inflammatory activities of extract of the leaves of *Sphenocentrum jollyannum* Pierre. J Applied Life Sci Int 2018; 18(4): 1-9.
[http://dx.doi.org/10.9734/JALSI/2018/34251]

[16]   Olorunnisola OS, Afolayan AJ. *In vivo* antioxidant and biochemical evaluation of *Sphenocentrum jollyanum* leaf extract in *P. berghei* infected mice. Pak J Pharm Sci 2013; 26(3): 445-50.
[PMID: 23625415]

[17]   Raji Y, Fadare OO, Adisa RA, Salami SA. Comprehensive assessment of the effect of *Sphenocentrum jollyanum* root extract on male reproductive activity in albino rats. Reprod Med Biol 2006; 5(4): 283-92.
[http://dx.doi.org/10.1111/j.1447-0578.2006.00154.x] [PMID: 29699257]

[18]   Harborne JB. Phytochemical methods A guide to modern technique of plant analysis. London: Chapman and Hall, Thompson Science 1973.

[19]   Sofowora AE. Medicinal plants and traditional medicine in Africa. 2nd ed., Ibadan, Nigeria: Spectrum Book Ltd 1993.

[20]   Pearson D. The chemical analysis of foods. 7th ed., New York: Edinburgh, Churchill Livingstone 1976.

[21]   Edeoga HO, Okwu DE, Mbaebie BO. Phytochemical constituents of some Nigerian medicinal plants. Afr J Biotechnol 2005; 4(7): 685-8.
[http://dx.doi.org/10.5897/AJB2005.000-3127]

[22]   Gould AN, Penny CB, Patel CC, Candy GP. Enhanced cutaneous wound healing by *Senecio*

serratuloides (Asteraceae/Compositae) in a pig model. S Afr J Bot 2015; 100: 63-8. [http://dx.doi.org/10.1016/j.sajb.2015.05.006]

[23] Bolton S, Bon C. Pharmaceutical Statistics: Practical and clinical applications. 4th ed., New York: Marcek Derker Inc 2004.

[24] Rieger S, Zhao H, Martin P, Abe K, Lisse TS. The role of nuclear hormone receptors in cutaneous wound repair. Cell Biochem Funct 2015; 33(1): 1-13. [http://dx.doi.org/10.1002/cbf.3086] [PMID: 25529612]

[25] Yabkowitz R, Meyer S, Black T, Elliott G, Merewether LA, Yamane HK. Inflammatory cytokines and vascular endothelial growth factor stimulate the release of soluble tie receptor from human endothelial cells *via* metalloprotease activation. Blood 1999; 93(6): 1969-79. [http://dx.doi.org/10.1182/blood.V93.6.1969.406k14_1969_1979] [PMID: 10068670]

[26] Ossovskaya VS, Bunnett NW. Protease-activated receptors: contribution to physiology and disease. Physiol Rev 2004; 84(2): 579-621. [http://dx.doi.org/10.1152/physrev.00028.2003] [PMID: 15044683]

[27] Schneider LA, Korber A, Grabbe S, Dissemond J. Influence of pH on wound-healing: a new perspective for wound-therapy? Arch Dermatol Res 2007; 298(9): 413-20. [http://dx.doi.org/10.1007/s00403-006-0713-x] [PMID: 17091276]

[28] Adongbede EM, Wisdom EO. Screening of some Nigerian medicinal plants for anti-candida activity. Amer J Drug Disc Dev 2013; 3: 60-71. [http://dx.doi.org/10.3923/ajdd.2013.60.71]

[29] Su X, Liu X, Wang S, *et al.* Wound-healing promoting effect of total tannins from *Entada phaseoloides* (L.) Merr. in rats. Burns 2017; 43(4): 830-8. [http://dx.doi.org/10.1016/j.burns.2016.10.010] [PMID: 28040363]

[30] Srivastava S, Yadav SKS, Chowdhury AR, Thombare N, Mitra P. Evaluation of wound healing properties of tannin isolated from Butea gum. Multilogic in Science 2018; 8(A): 368-9.

[31] Porras-Reyes BH, Lewis WH, Roman J, Simchowitz L, Mustoe TA. Enhancement of wound healing by the alkaloid taspine defining mechanism of action. Proc Soc Exp Biol Med 1993; 203(1): 18-25. [http://dx.doi.org/10.3181/00379727-203-43567] [PMID: 8386382]

[32] Fetse JP, Kyekyeku JO, Dueve E, Mensah KB. Wound healing activity of total alkaloidal extract of the root bark of *Alstonia boonei* (Apocyanaceae). Br J Pharm Res 2014; 4(23): 2642-52. [http://dx.doi.org/10.9734/BJPR/2014/13952]

[33] Tang T, Yin L, Yang J, Shan G. Emodin, an anthraquinone derivative from *Rheum officinale* Baill, enhances cutaneous wound healing in rats. Eur J Pharmacol 2007; 567(3): 177-85. [http://dx.doi.org/10.1016/j.ejphar.2007.02.033] [PMID: 17540366]

[34] Vaisberg AJ, Milla M, Planas MC, *et al.* Taspine is the cicatrizant principle in Sangre de Grado extracted from *Croton lechleri.* Planta Med 1989; 55(2): 140-3. [http://dx.doi.org/10.1055/s-2006-961907] [PMID: 2748730]

SUBJECT INDEX

A

Abortion 87
  spontaneous 25, 26, 27, 28
Abortions, induced 87
ABTS Radical Scavenging Assay 96
Acid 16, 68, 70, 75, 78, 84, 85, 87, 88, 89, 90, 91, 93, 97, 98, 99, 100
  acetic 88, 90, 98
  arachidonic 97
  aristolochic (AA) 16, 84, 85, 88, 89, 90, 93, 97, 99, 100
  caprylic 91
  citric 78
  glycolic 70, 75
  hydrocyanic 68
  lauric 91
  linoleic 91, 99
  linolenic 91, 97
  nitrophenanthrene carboxylic 88
  oleic 97, 98
  palmitic 85, 90, 97
  palmitoleic 97
  tannic 85, 87
Activities 37, 40, 41, 43, 48, 57, 67, 76, 91, 97, 98, 100, 113
  analgesic 37, 41, 43, 113
  anti-atherothrombosis 43
  antidiabetic 98
  anti-diarrheal 40
  antilithiasic 67, 76
  antimicrobial 91, 97
  anti-nociceptive 40
  antipsoriatic 57
  cytotoxic 97
  efficient 98
  enzymatic 97
  inhibiting disaccharidase 98
  inhibitory 95
  moderate anti-viral 48
  nephrotoxic 100

  thrombolytic 41
Acute 41, 96, 100
  hepatotoxicity 96, 100
  myocardial infarction 41
Aeromonas hydrophila 40
Agar diffusion method 94
Age 26, 27, 63
  gestational 26
  reproductive 27
Agents 41, 47, 78
  antilithogenic 78
  causative 40
  selective anti-CHIKV 47
  thrombolytic 41
Aggregation process 79
Agricultural soils 20
Allergic symptoms 60
Allium sativum 69, 70, 78
Alteration electrostatic hydrogen 99
Analgesic effect 42
Andrographis paniculata 48
Andrographolide 48, 49
Antibacterial 88, 89, 91, 97
  activities 88, 91, 97
  and antifungal activities 97
  properties 89
Anticancer properties 88
Anti-CHIKV drugs 46
Antidiabetic herbal medicines 1, 2, 3, 4, 7, 8, 10
Anti-diabetic herbal preparations (ADHP) 15, 16, 17, 18, 19, 20
Anti-diarrheal 40, 43
  effect 43
  activity 40
Antifungal Activities 97
Anti-inflammatory
  activities 40, 57, 65, 91, 99
  condition 57
  effect 40, 65, 99
Antilithiasic properties 68, 79
Antilithiatic 70

www.ingramcontent.com/pod-product-compliance
Lightning Source LLC
Chambersburg PA
CBHW041715210326
41598CB00007B/662